Sexual Health Information for Teens

Second Edition

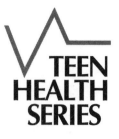

TEEN HEALTH SERIES

Second Edition

Sexual Health Information for Teens

Health Tips about Sexual Development, Reproduction, Contraception, and Sexually Transmitted Infections

Including Facts about Puberty, Sexuality, Birth Control, Chlamydia, Gonorrhea, Herpes, Human Papillomavirus, Syphilis, and More

◆

Edited by Sandra Augustyn Lawton

Omnigraphics

P.O. Box 31-1640, Detroit, MI 48231

Bibliographic Note

Because this page cannot legibly accommodate all the copyright notices, the Bibliographic Note portion of the Preface constitutes an extension of the copyright notice.

Edited by Sandra Augustyn Lawton

Teen Health Series

Karen Bellenir, *Managing Editor*
David A. Cooke, M.D., *Medical Consultant*
Elizabeth Collins, *Research and Permissions Coordinator*
Cherry Stockdale, *Permissions Assistant*
EdIndex, Services for Publishers, *Indexers*

* * *

Omnigraphics, Inc.
Matthew P. Barbour, *Senior Vice President*
Kevin M. Hayes, *Operations Manager*

* * *

Peter E. Ruffner, *Publisher*

Copyright © 2008 Omnigraphics, Inc.

ISBN 978-0-7808-1010-5

Library of Congress Cataloging-in-Publication Data

Sexual health information for teens : health tips about sexual development, reproduction, contraception, and sexually transmitted infections including facts about puberty, sexuality, birth control, chlamydia, gonorrhea, herpes, human papillomavirus, syphilis, and more / edited by Sandra Augustyn Lawton. -- 2nd ed.
  p. cm.
  Includes bibliographical references and index.
  Summary: "Provides basic consumer health information for teens about puberty, sexuality, reproductive health, contraception, and disease prevention. Includes index, resource information, and recommendation for further reading"--Provided by publisher.
  ISBN 978-0-7808-1010-5 (hardcover : alk. paper) 1. Teenagers--Health and hygiene. 2. Hygiene, Sexual. 3. Reproductive health. 4. Puberty. 5. Sexually transmitted diseases--Prevention. 6. Sex instruction for teenagers. I. Lawton, Sandra Augustyn.
  RA777.S47 2008
  613.90835--dc22

2007052454

Table of Contents

Preface ix

Part One: What To Expect As Your Body Exits Childhood

Chapter 1—Growing Up 3

Chapter 2—What Are Hormones? 7

Chapter 3—Puberty: An Overview 17

Chapter 4—What Happens To Girls At Puberty? 25

Chapter 5—What Happens To Guys At Puberty? 29

Chapter 6—When Puberty Starts Early 35

Chapter 7—When Puberty Starts Late 39

Chapter 8—Surviving Puberty: Moods And Emotions 45

Part Two: Protecting Your Sexual Health

Chapter 9—Seven Steps To Sexual Health 51

Chapter 10—Finding The Right Clinic And The Services
            They Offer 55

Chapter 11—Facts On American Teens' Sexual And
            Reproductive Health 61

Chapter 12—Talking With Your Parents About Sex 65

Chapter 13—How Do You Know When You're Ready For Sex? 69

Chapter 14—Abstinence: A Personal Choice 79

Chapter 15—Masturbation 83

Chapter 16—Oral Sex: Is It Really Sex? 87

Chapter 17—Sexual Orientation And Homosexuality 91

Chapter 18—Transgender Individuals And Gender Identity 97

Chapter 19—Sexuality In The Mass Media: How To View The
              Media Critically 101

Chapter 20—Rape And Date Rape: What You Should Know 107

Chapter 21—Protecting Yourself From Online Sexual Predators 111

Part Three: For Girls Only

Chapter 22—The Female Reproductive System: An Overview 119

Chapter 23—Menstruation And The Menstrual Cycle 127

Chapter 24—Premenstrual Syndrome 137

Chapter 25—Douching 141

Chapter 26—First Visit To The Gynecologist 145

Chapter 27—Pap Test 151

Chapter 28—Breast Self-Exam 157

Chapter 29—Facts About Breast Cancer 163

Chapter 30—Teens And Breast Implants 169

Chapter 31—Toxic Shock Syndrome 173

Chapter 32—Urinary Tract Infection 177

Chapter 33—Vaginal Yeast Infections And Bacterial Vaginosis 181

Chapter 34—Pelvic Inflammatory Disease 189

Chapter 35—Endometriosis 195

Chapter 36—Turner Syndrome 201

Part Four: For Guys Only

Chapter 37—The Male Reproductive System: An Overview 209

Chapter 38—Circumcision 217

Chapter 39—Is My Penis Normal? 221

Chapter 40—Wet Dreams: A Guide To Nocturnal Emissions 223

Chapter 41—Testicular Self-Exam 225

Chapter 42—Testicular Cancer 227

Chapter 43—Testicular Injuries 233

Chapter 44—Guys And Enlarged Breasts: Gynecomastia 237

Chapter 45—Klinefelter Syndrome 239

Part Five: Pregnancy Prevention

Chapter 46—Teen Pregnancy Facts 245

Chapter 47—Pregnancy Prevention Programs: Abstinence
Versus Comprehensive Sex Education 249

Chapter 48—Rhythm Method 257

Chapter 49—Male Condom 261

Chapter 50—Female Condom 267

Chapter 51—Diaphragm, Cervical Cap, And Cervical Shield 271

Chapter 52—Contraceptive Sponge 281

Chapter 53—Oral Contraceptives 283

Chapter 54—The Patch 289

Chapter 55—The Shot 299

Chapter 56—Intrauterine Devices And Systems 303

Chapter 57—Vaginal Ring 309

Chapter 58—Sterilization 317

Chapter 59—Emergency Contraception 323

Part Six: Sexually Transmitted Diseases

Chapter 60—Questions And Answers About Sexually
  Transmitted Diseases 331

Chapter 61—Chlamydia 335

Chapter 62—Genital Herpes 339

Chapter 63—Gonorrhea 345

Chapter 64—Hepatitis B 349

Chapter 65—Human Immunodeficiency Virus (HIV)
  And Acquired Immune Deficiency Syndrome
  (AIDS) 355

Chapter 66—Human Papillomavirus 363

Chapter 67—Molluscum Contagiosum 371

Chapter 68—Nongonococcal Urethritis 375

Chapter 69—Pubic Lice 381

Chapter 70—Scabies 385

Chapter 71—Syphilis 389

Chapter 72—Trichomoniasis 395

Part Seven: If You Need More Information

Chapter 73—Resources For Additional Information About
  Sexual Development And Sexually Transmitted
  Diseases 401

Chapter 74—Additional Reading About Sexuality And
  Sexual Health 407

Index 415

Preface

About This Book

As they mature and prepare for adulthood, teens face many academic and social challenges. In addition, they must also deal with developing bodies, sexual pressures from peers, and alluring media messages. According to statistics gathered in 2005 by the National Center for Chronic Disease Prevention and Health Promotion, 47% of high school students reported having had sexual intercourse; 14% reported having had four or more sex partners. Irrespective of whether and when teens choose to enter sexual relationships, they need accurate information about how their choices can affect their health.

Sexual Health Information for Teens, Second Edition offers updated facts about the sexual issues today's teens face. It describes reproductive anatomy and the physical and emotional changes that accompany puberty and emerging sexuality, including sensitive issues such as contraception, masturbation, oral sex, and sexual orientation. It offers facts about activities that can put teens at risk for unplanned pregnancies and sexually transmitted diseases. The long-term consequences of untreated sexually transmitted infections and infections for which no cure currently exists—including cervical and other cancers, liver disease, pelvic inflammatory disease, and infertility—are also discussed. The book concludes with a directory of resources for further information and suggestions for additional reading.

How To Use This Book

This book is divided into parts and chapters. Parts focus on broad areas of interest; chapters are devoted to single topics within a part.

Part One: What To Expect As Your Body Exits Childhood explains that confusing time in life when a person's body becomes sexually mature—a process known as puberty. It talks about male and female hormones, describes the specific changes that affect boys and girls in different ways, and provides facts about the mental changes and mood swings that often accompany puberty's physical transformations.

Part Two: Protecting Your Sexual Health includes information to help teens develop an awareness of issues that can impact their ability to enjoy their sexuality for a lifetime. It discusses developing self-awareness, and talks about medical privacy and confidentiality. One chapter offers suggestions for communicating with parents about sexual issues. The part concludes with facts to help teens protect themselves from rape and online sexual predators.

Part Three: For Girls Only begins with an anatomical review of the female reproductive system. It addresses concerns girls often have about the menstrual cycle, douching, and routine gynecological care. It also offers facts about medical issues that are more commonly associated with females, including breast cancer, toxic shock syndrome, and urinary tract infection.

Part Four: For Guys Only begins with an anatomical review of the male reproductive system. It addresses concerns boys often have about circumcision, penile development, nocturnal emissions, routine urological care, and testicular injuries. It concludes with information about gynecomastia (enlarged breasts in males) and Klinefelter syndrome, a condition in males who have an extra X chromosome.

Part Five: Pregnancy Prevention offers facts about teen pregnancy and pregnancy prevention programs, including abstinence-based programs and comprehensive sex education programs. It explains different kinds of contraceptives and how to use them correctly. It also provides information on their reliability and whether or not they protect against sexually transmitted diseases.

Part Six: Sexually Transmitted Diseases includes information about chlamydia, gonorrhea, herpes, hepatitis B, syphilis, and other diseases that are spread by sexual contact. It describes how different types of infections—bacterial, viral, and fungal—are transmitted, the steps that can be taken to avoid them, symptoms that may accompany infection, available treatments, and the long-term consequences associated with untreated infections and diseases for which no cure currently exists.

Part Seven: If You Need More Information offers a directory of resources and suggestions for additional information about sexual development, sexual health, and sexually transmitted diseases.

Bibliographic Note

This volume contains documents and excerpts from publications issued by the following government agencies: Centers for Disease Control and Prevention (CDC); National Cancer Institute (NCI); National Institute of Allergy and Infectious Diseases (NIAID); National Institute of Child Health and Human Development (NICHD); National Institute of Diabetes and Digestive and Kidney Diseases (NIDDK); National Institutes of Health (NIH); National Women's Health Information Center (NWHIC); Substance Abuse and Mental Health Services Administration (SAMHSA); U.S. Department of Veterans Affairs; U.S. Food and Drug Administration (FDA); and the United States Senate.

In addition, this volume contains copyrighted documents and articles produced by the following organizations: A.D.A.M., Inc.; Advocates for Youth; American Board of Obstetrics and Gynecology, Inc.; American Pregnancy Association; American Psychological Association; American Social Health Association; American Society of Health-System Pharmacists, Inc.; AVERT; Cincinnati Children's Hospital Medical Center; Emory University; Family Planning Association of Western Australia; Alan Guttmacher Institute; Hormone Foundation; Henry J. Kaiser Family Foundation; Massachusetts Medical Society; Medical Institute for Sexual Health; Nemours Foundation; Planned Parenthood Federation of America, Inc.; Planned Parenthood of New York City; Province of British Columbia; Society of Obstetricians and Gynaecologists of Canada; State of California Department of Health, Cancer Detection Section; University of California, Santa Barbara; University of Florida Counseling Center; University of Ottawa Health Services; Washington State University Health and Wellness Services; Women's College Hospital.

Full citation information is provided on the first page of each chapter. Every effort has been made to secure all necessary rights to reprint the copyrighted material. If any omissions have been made, please contact Omnigraphics to make corrections for future editions.

The photograph on the front cover is from Iryna Kurhan/Shutterstock.com.

Acknowledgements

In addition to the organizations listed above, special thanks are due to the *Teen Health Series* research and permissions coordinator, Elizabeth Collins, and to its managing editor, Karen Bellenir.

About the *Teen Health Series*

At the request of librarians serving today's young adults, the *Teen Health Series* was developed as a specially focused set of volumes within Omnigraphics' *Health Reference Series*. Each volume deals comprehensively with a topic selected according to the needs and interests of people in middle school and high school.

Teens seeking preventive guidance, information about disease warning signs, medical statistics, and risk factors for health problems will find answers to their questions in the *Teen Health Series*. The *Series*, however, is not intended to serve as a tool for diagnosing illness, in prescribing treatments, or as a substitute for the physician/patient relationship. All people concerned about medical symptoms or the possibility of disease are encouraged to seek professional care from an appropriate health care provider.

If there is a topic you would like to see addressed in a future volume of the *Teen Health Series*, please write to:

Editor
Teen Health Series
Omnigraphics, Inc.
P.O. Box 31-1640
Detroit, MI 48231

A Note about Spelling and Style

Teen Health Series editors use *Stedman's Medical Dictionary* as an authority for questions related to the spelling of medical terms and the *Chicago Manual of Style* for questions related to grammatical structures, punctuation, and other editorial concerns. Consistent adherence is not always possible, however, because the individual volumes within the *Series* include many documents from a wide variety of different producers and copyright holders, and the editor's primary goal is to present material from each source as accurately as is possible following the terms specified by each document's producer. This sometimes means that information in different chapters or sections may follow other guidelines and alternate spelling authorities. For example, occasionally a copyright holder may require that eponymous terms be shown in possessive forms (Crohn's disease *vs.* Crohn disease) or that British spelling norms be retained (leukaemia *vs.* leukemia).

Locating Information within the *Teen Health Series*

The *Teen Health Series* contains a wealth of information about a wide variety of medical topics. As the *Series* continues to grow in size and scope, locating the precise information needed by a specific student may become more challenging. To address this concern, information about books within the *Teen Health Series* is included in *A Contents Guide to the Health Reference Series*. The *Contents Guide* presents an extensive list of more than 13,000 diseases, treatments, and other topics of general interest compiled from the Tables of Contents and major index headings from the books of the *Teen Health Series* and *Health Reference Series*. To access *A Contents Guide to the Health Reference Series*, visit www.healthreferenceseries.com.

Our Advisory Board

We would like to thank the following advisory board members for providing guidance to the development of this *Series*:

Dr. Lynda Baker, Associate Professor of Library and Information Science, Wayne State University, Detroit, MI

Nancy Bulgarelli, William Beaumont Hospital Library, Royal Oak, MI

Karen Imarisio, Bloomfield Township Public Library, Bloomfield Township, MI

Karen Morgan, Mardigian Library, University of Michigan-Dearborn, Dearborn, MI

Rosemary Orlando, St. Clair Shores Public Library, St. Clair Shores, MI

Medical Consultant

Medical consultation services are provided to the *Teen Health Series* editors by David A. Cooke, M.D. Dr. Cooke is a graduate of Brandeis University, and he received his M.D. degree from the University of Michigan. He completed residency training at the University of Wisconsin Hospital and Clinics. He is board-certified in internal medicine. Dr. Cooke currently works as part of the University of Michigan Health System and practices in Ann Arbor, MI. In his free time, he enjoys writing, science fiction, and spending time with his family.

Part One

What To Expect As Your Body Exits Childhood

Chapter 1

Growing Up

Since your last birthday, a lot of things have changed. For one, you're much smarter than you were last year. That's obvious.

But there might have been some other changes—ones that you weren't ready for. Perhaps you've sprouted several inches above everyone else in class. Or maybe they all did the sprouting, and you feel too short. Maybe you haven't gained a pound and you feel like a feather on the seesaw, or maybe you can't fit into your favorite pair of jeans. And now you're looking in the mirror, thinking only one thing: Am I normal?

Everybody's Different

First of all, what's normal? There's no one normal. Otherwise, the world would be full of a lot of abnormal people. The next time you go to the mall, take a look around. You'll see tall people, short people, and people with broad shoulders, little feet, big stomachs, long fingers, stubby legs, and skinny arms . . . you get the idea.

You can change your hairstyle or put on a new hat, but the way you look isn't entirely under your control. Your looks were largely determined by your

About This Chapter: Information in this chapter is from "I'm Growing Up—But Am I Normal?" This information was provided by KidsHealth, one of the largest resources online for medically reviewed health information written for parents, kids, and teens. For more articles like this one, visit www.KidsHealth.org, or www.TeensHealth.org. © 2005 The Nemours Foundation.

parents. When your parents created you, they passed on their genes—a kind of special code—and those genes helped to decide your size and shape, your eye color and hair texture, even whether you have freckles.

Small Or Tall

Height is just one of the thousands of features your genes decide. In fact, because you have two parents, your genes act like a referee, giving you a height that usually lands somewhere between the height of each parent. If both your parents are tall, then most likely you will be tall, too, but if you have questions about how tall you're going to be, ask your doctor if he or she can help you figure it out.

But genes don't decide everything. For example, eating an unhealthy diet can keep you from growing to your full potential. Getting plenty of sleep, enough exercise, and nutrients will help you grow just like you should.

No doubt you're wondering how fast you should grow. It depends. There's no perfect or right amount. On average, kids grow about two inches (six centimeters) a year between age three and when they start puberty (when your body starts changing and becoming more grown up).

Your doctor will know how your growth has been going over the years. Two centimeters here and two inches there are not nearly as important as the height you're at now, how you've been growing up to this point, and what other changes your body may be going through.

Don't be scared if you seem to have grown a lot in a very short time. Everyone has a growth spurt during puberty. The average age for starting puberty is about 10 for girls and about 11 for boys. But it can be earlier or later—between 7 and 13 for girls and 9 and 15 for boys.

Weighing In

Weight can vary a lot, too, from kid to kid. It's tempting to compare yourself to your friends. But kids often weigh more or less than their friends and are still considered normal. TV and magazines might make us think our bodies should weigh and look a certain way, but in real life, there are a lot of differences.

Some kids worry so much about their weight that they try unhealthy and dangerous things to change it. The best way to have a healthy weight is to eat right and get a lot of playtime (exercise).

What To Do If You're Worried

If you have concerns about your weight—or how your body is changing—talk it over with a parent or your doctor. The doctor can tell you if anything is wrong. But most likely, your one-of-a-kind body is growing just like it's supposed to.

♣ **It's A Fact!!**
You'll usually begin to notice that you're growing faster about a year or so after your body starts to show the first changes of puberty—girls will develop breasts and a boy's penis and testicles will get bigger.

Chapter 2

What Are Hormones?

The Endocrine System

The endocrine system is one of the body's main systems for communicating, controlling, and coordinating the body's work. It works with the nervous system, reproductive system, kidneys, gut, liver, and fat to help maintain and control the following:

- body energy levels

- reproduction

- growth and development

- internal balance of body systems, called homeostasis

- responses to surroundings, stress, and injury

The endocrine system accomplishes these tasks via a network of glands and organs that produce, store, and secrete certain hormones. Hormones are special chemicals that move into body fluid after they are made by one cell or a group of cells. Hormones cause an effect on other cells or tissues of the body.

About This Chapter: Information under the heading "The Endocrine System" is from "Endo 101: The Endocrine System." Text under the heading "Endocrine Glands" is from "Endocrine Glands." © 2005 The Hormone Foundation. Reprinted with permission. For additional information, visit www.hormone.org.

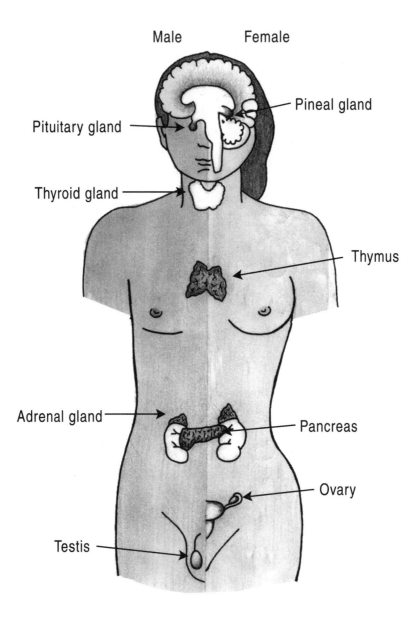

Figure 2.1. Endocrine Organs of the Human Body (Source: Surveillance, Epidemiology and End Results, National Cancer Institute; redrawn for Omnigraphics by Alison DeKleine, 2007.)

Endocrine glands make hormones that are used inside the body. Other glands make substances, like saliva, reach the outside of the body. Endocrine glands and endocrine-related organs are like factories. They produce and store hormones and release them as needed. When the body needs these substances, the bloodstream carries the hormones to specific targets. These targets may be organs, tissues, or cells. To function normally, the body needs glands that work correctly, a blood supply that works well to move hormones through the body to their target points, receptor places on the target cells for the hormones to do their work, and a system for controlling how hormones are produced and used.

What could go wrong? Endocrine disorders happen when one or more of the endocrine systems in your body are not working well. Hormones may be released in amounts that are too great or too small for the body to work normally. There may not be enough receptors, or binding sites, for the hormones so that they can direct the work that needs to be done. There could be a problem with the system regulating the hormones in the bloodstream, or the body may have difficulty controlling hormone levels because of problems clearing hormones from the blood. For example, a person's liver or kidneys may not be working well, and this might keep too high a hormone level in the bloodstream.

✤ It's A Fact!!

If you or your primary care physician suspects that you have an endocrine disorder, you may need a specialist called an endocrinologist. An endocrinologist is a specially trained doctor who diagnoses and treats diseases that affect your glands and hormone levels (endocrine system). They know how to treat conditions, which are often complex and involve many systems and structures within your body. Your regular doctor refers you to an endocrinologist when you have a problem with your endocrine system.

Source: Excerpted from "Endo 101: The Endocrine System," © 2005 The Hormone Foundation.

Endocrine Glands

Pituitary Gland

The pituitary gland is sometimes called the "master gland" because of its great influence on the other body organs. Its function is complex and important for overall well-being.

The pituitary gland is divided into two parts, front (anterior) and back (posterior).

The anterior pituitary produces several hormones, and they are as follows:

- **Prolactin Or PRL:** PRL stimulates milk production from a woman's breasts after childbirth and can affect sex hormone levels from the ovaries in women and the testes in men.

- **Growth Hormone Or GH:** GH stimulates growth in childhood and is important for maintaining a healthy body composition. In adults, it is also important for maintaining muscle mass and bone mass. It can affect fat distribution in the body.

- **Adrenocorticotropin Or ACTH:** ACTH stimulates production of cortisol by the adrenal glands. Cortisol, a so-called "stress hormone," is vital to survival. It helps maintain blood pressure and blood glucose levels.

- **Thyroid-Stimulating Hormone Or TSH:** TSH stimulates the thyroid gland to make thyroid hormones, which, in turn, control (regulate) the body's metabolism, energy, growth and development, and nervous system activity.

- **Luteinizing Hormone Or LH:** LH regulates testosterone in men and estrogen in women.

- **Follicle-Stimulating Hormone Or FSH:** FSH promotes sperm production in men and stimulates the ovaries to release eggs (ovulate) in women. LH and FSH work together to allow normal function of the ovaries or testes.

The posterior pituitary produces two hormones, and they are as follows:

- **Oxytocin:** Oxytocin causes milk letdown in nursing mothers and contractions during childbirth.

- **Antidiuretic Hormone Or ADH:** ADH, also called vasopressin, is stored in the back part of the pituitary gland and regulates water balance. If this hormone is not secreted properly, this can lead to problems of sodium (salt) and water balance, and could also affect the kidneys so that they do not work as well.

Hypothalamus

The hypothalamus is part of the brain that lies just above the pituitary gland. It releases hormones that start and stop the release of pituitary hormones. The hypothalamus controls hormone production in the pituitary gland through several "releasing" hormones. Some of these are growth hormone-releasing hormone, or (controls GH release); thyrotropin-releasing hormone, or TRH (controls TSH release); and corticotropin-releasing hormone, or CRH (controls ACTH release). Gonadotropin-releasing hormone (GnRH) tells the pituitary gland to make luteinizing hormone (LH) and follicle-stimulating hormone (FSH), which are important for normal puberty.

♣ It's A Fact!!

In response to over- or underproduction of pituitary hormones, the target glands affected by these hormones can produce too many or too few hormones of their own. For example, too much growth hormone can cause gigantism, or excessive growth, while too little GH may cause dwarfism, or very short stature.

Source: Excerpted from "Endocrine Glands," © 2005 The Hormone Foundation.

Thymus

The thymus is a gland needed early in life for normal immune function. It is very large just after a child is born and weighs its greatest when a child reaches puberty. Then its tissue is replaced by fat. The thymus gland secretes hormones called humoral factors. These hormones help to develop the lymphoid system, which is a system throughout the body that help it to reach a mature immune response in cells to protect them from invading bodies, like bacteria.

Pineal Gland

Scientists are still learning how the pineal gland works. They have found one hormone so far that is produced by this gland: melatonin. Melatonin may stop the action of (inhibit) the hormones that produce gonadotropin, which causes the ovaries and testes to develop and function. It may also help to control sleep patterns.

Testes

Males have twin reproductive glands, called testes that produce the hormone testosterone. Testosterone helps a boy develop and then maintain his sexual traits. During puberty, testosterone helps to bring about the physical changes that turn a boy into an adult male, such as growth of the penis and testes, growth of facial and pubic hair, deepening of the voice, increase in muscle mass and strength, and increase in height. Throughout adult life, testosterone helps maintain sex drive, sperm production, male hair patterns, muscle mass, and bone mass.

Testicular cancer, which is the most common form of cancer for males between ages 15 and 35, may need to be treated by surgical removal of one or both testicles. The resulting decrease or absence of testosterone may cause decreased sexual drive, impotence, altered body image, and other symptoms.

Ovaries

The two most important hormones of a woman's twin reproductive glands, the ovaries, are estrogen and progesterone. These hormones are responsible for developing and maintaining female sexual traits, as well as maintaining a pregnancy. Along with the pituitary gonadotropins (FH and LSH), they also control the menstrual cycle. The ovaries also produce inhibin, a protein that curbs (inhibits) the release of follicle-stimulating hormone from the anterior pituitary and helps control egg development.

The most common change in the ovarian hormones is caused by the start of menopause, part of the normal aging process. It also can occur when ovaries are removed surgically. Loss of ovarian function means loss of estrogen, which can lead to hot flashes, thinning vaginal tissue, lack of menstrual periods, mood changes and bone loss, or osteoporosis.

A condition called polycystic ovary syndrome (PCOS) is caused by over-production of male hormones in females. PCOS can affect menstrual cycles, fertility, and hormone levels, as well as cause acne, facial hair growth, and male pattern balding.

Thyroid

The thyroid is a small gland inside the neck, located in front of your breathing airway (trachea) and below your Adam's apple. The thyroid hormones control your metabolism, which is the body's ability to break down food and store it as energy and the ability to break down food into waste products with a release of energy in the process. The thyroid produces two hormones, T3 (called triiodothyronine) and T4 (called thyroxine).

Thyroid disorders result from too little or too much thyroid hormone. Symptoms of hypothyroidism (too little hormone) include decreased energy, slow heart rate, dry skin, constipation, and feeling cold all the time. In children, hypothyroidism most commonly leads to slowed growth. Infants born with hypothyroidism can have delayed development and mental retardation if not treated. In adults, this disorder often causes weight gain. An enlarged thyroid, or goiter, may develop.

Hyperthyroidism (too much hormone) may result in exophthalmic goiter, or Graves disease. Symptoms include anxiety, fast heart rate, diarrhea, and weight loss. An enlarged thyroid gland (goiter) and swelling behind the eyes that causes the eyes to push forward, or bulge out, are common.

Adrenal Glands

Each adrenal gland is actually two endocrine organs. The outer portion is called the adrenal cortex. The inner portion is called the adrenal medulla. The hormones of the adrenal cortex are essential for life. The hormones of the adrenal medulla are not.

The adrenal cortex produces glucocorticoids (such as cortisol) that help the body control blood sugar, increase the burning of protein and fat, and respond to stressors like fever, major illness, and injury. The mineralocorticoids (such as aldosterone) control blood volume and help to regulate blood pressure by acting on the kidneys to help them hold onto enough sodium and water. The adrenal cortex also produces some sex hormones, which are important for some secondary sex characteristics in both men and women.

Two important disorders caused by problems with the adrenal cortex are Cushing syndrome (too much cortisol) and Addison disease (too little cortisol).

The adrenal medulla produces epinephrine (adrenaline), which is secreted by nerve endings and increases the heart rate, opens airways to improve oxygen intake, and increases blood flow to muscles, usually when a person is scared, excited, or under stress.

Norepinephrine also is made by the adrenal medulla, but this hormone is more related to maintaining normal activities as opposed to emergency reactions. Too much norepinephrine can cause high blood pressure.

Parathyroid

Located behind the thyroid gland are four tiny parathyroid glands. These make hormones that help control calcium and phosphorous levels in the body. The parathyroid glands are necessary for proper bone development. In response to too little calcium in the diet, the parathyroid glands make parathyroid hormone, or PTH, that takes calcium from bones so that it will be available in the blood for nerve conduction and muscle contraction.

If the parathyroids are removed during a thyroid operation, low blood calcium will result in symptoms such as irregular heartbeat, muscle spasms, tingling in the hands and feet, and possibly difficulty breathing. A tumor or chronic illness can cause too much secretion of PTH and lead to bone pain, kidney stones, increased urination, muscle weakness, and fatigue.

Pancreas

The pancreas is a large gland behind your stomach that helps the body to maintain healthy blood sugar (glucose) levels. The pancreas secretes insulin, a hormone that helps glucose move from the blood into the cells where it is used for energy. The pancreas also secretes glucagon when the blood sugar is low. Glucagon tells the liver to release glucose, stored in the liver as glycogen, into the bloodstream.

Diabetes, an imbalance of blood sugar levels, is the major disorder of the pancreas. Diabetes occurs when the pancreas does not produce enough insulin (Type 1) or the body is resistant to the insulin in the blood (Type 2). Without enough insulin to keep glucose moving through the metabolic process, the blood glucose level rises too high.

In Type 1 diabetes, a patient must take insulin shots. In Type 2 diabetes, a patient may not necessarily need insulin and can sometimes control blood sugar levels with exercise, diet, and other medications.

A condition called hyperinsulinism (HI) is caused by too much insulin and leads to hypoglycemia (low blood sugar). The inherited form, called congenital HI, causes severe hypoglycemia in infancy. Sometimes it can be treated with medication but often requires surgical removal of part or all of the pancreas. An insulin-secreting tumor of the pancreas, or insulinoma, is a less common cause of hypoglycemia. Symptoms of low blood sugar include anxiety, sweating, increased heart rate, weakness, hunger, and light-headedness. Low blood sugar stimulates release of epinephrine, glucagon, and growth hormone, which help to return the blood sugar to normal.

Chapter 3

Puberty: An Overview

OK, so it's a funny word ... but what is puberty, anyway? Puberty is the name for when your body begins to develop and change. During puberty, your body will grow faster than any other time in your life, except for when you were an infant. Back then, your body was growing rapidly, and you were learning new things—you'll be doing these things and much more during puberty. Except this time, you won't have diapers or a rattle, and you'll have to dress yourself.

It's good to know about the changes that come along with puberty before they happen, and it's really important to remember that everybody goes through it. No matter where you live, whether you're a guy or a girl, or whether you like hip-hop or country music, you will experience the changes that occur during puberty. No two people are exactly alike. But one thing all adults have in common is they made it through puberty.

Time To Change

When your body reaches a certain age, your brain releases a special hormone that starts the changes of puberty. It's called gonadotropin-releasing hormone, or GnRH for short. When GnRH reaches the pituitary gland (a

About This Chapter: Information in this chapter is from "Everything You Wanted to Know About Puberty." This information was provided by TeensHealth, one of the largest resources online for medically reviewed health information written for parents, kids, and teens. For more articles like this one, visit www.TeensHealth.org, or www.KidsHealth.org. © 2007 The Nemours Foundation.

pea-shaped gland that sits just under the brain), this gland releases into the bloodstream two more puberty hormones: luteinizing hormone (LH for short) and follicle-stimulating hormone (FSH for short). Guys and girls have both of these hormones in their bodies. And depending on whether you're a guy or a girl, these hormones go to work on different parts of the body.

For guys, these hormones travel through the blood and give the testes the signal to begin the production of testosterone and sperm. Testosterone is the hormone that causes most of the changes in a guy's body during puberty. Sperm cells must be produced for men to reproduce.

In girls, FSH and LH target the ovaries, which contain eggs that have been there since birth. The hormones stimulate the ovaries to begin producing another hormone called estrogen. Estrogen, along with FSH and LH, causes a girl's body to mature and prepares her for pregnancy.

So that's what's really happening during puberty—it's all these new chemicals moving around inside your body, turning you from a teen into an adult with adult levels of hormones.

♣ It's A Fact!!

Puberty usually starts some time between age 8 and 13 in girls and 10 and 15 in guys. Some people start puberty a bit earlier or later, though. Each person is a little different, so everyone starts and goes through puberty on his or her body's own schedule. This is one of the reasons why some of your friends might still look like kids, whereas others look more like adults.

Source: © 2007 The Nemours Foundation.

It Doesn't Hurt . . . It's Just A Growth Spurt

"Spurt" is the word used to describe a short burst of activity, something that happens in a hurry. And a growth spurt is just that: Your body is growing, and it's happening really fast. When you enter puberty, it might seem like your sleeves are always getting shorter, and your pants always look like you're ready for a flood—that's because you're experiencing a major growth spurt. It lasts for about two to three years. When that growth spurt is at its peak, some people grow four or more inches in a year.

This growth during puberty will be the last time your body grows taller. After that, you will be at your adult height. But your height isn't the only thing that will be changing.

Taking Shape

As your body grows taller, it will change in other ways, too. You will gain weight, and as your body becomes heavier, you'll start to notice changes in its overall shape. Guys' shoulders will grow wider, and their bodies will become more muscular. Their voices will become deeper. For some guys, the breasts may grow a bit, but for most of them this growth goes away by the end of puberty.

Guys will notice other changes, too, like the lengthening and widening of the penis and the enlargement of the testes. All of these changes mean that their bodies are developing as expected during puberty.

Girls' bodies usually become curvier. They gain weight on their hips, and their breasts develop, starting with just a little swelling under the nipple. Sometimes one breast might develop more quickly than the other, but most of the time they soon even out. With all this growing and developing going on, girls will notice an increase in body fat and occasional soreness under the nipples as the breasts start to enlarge—and that's normal.

Gaining some weight is part of developing into a woman, and it's unhealthy for girls to go on a diet to try to stop this normal weight gain. If you ever have questions or concerns about your weight, talk it over with your doctor.

Usually about two to two and one-half years after girls' breasts start to develop, they get their first menstrual period. This is one more thing that lets a girl know puberty is progressing, and the puberty hormones have been doing their job. Girls have two ovaries, and each ovary holds thousands of eggs. During the menstrual cycle, one of the eggs comes out of an ovary and begins a trip through the fallopian tube, ending up in the uterus (the uterus is also called the womb).

Before the egg is released from the ovary, the uterus has been building up its lining with extra blood and tissue. If the egg is fertilized by a sperm cell, it stays in the uterus and grows into a baby, using that extra blood and tissue to keep it healthy and protected as it's developing.

Most of the time, though, the egg is only passing through. When the egg doesn't get fertilized, the uterus no longer needs the extra blood and tissue, so it leaves the body through the vagina as a menstrual period. A period usually lasts from five to seven days, and about two weeks after the start of the period a new egg is released, which marks the middle of each cycle.

Hair, Hair, Everywhere

Well, maybe not everywhere. But one of the first signs of puberty is hair growing where it didn't grow before. Guys and girls both begin to grow hair under their arms and in their pubic areas (on and around the genitals). It starts out looking light and sparse. Then as you go through puberty, it becomes longer, thicker, heavier, and darker. Eventually, guys also start to grow hair on their faces.

About Face

Another thing that comes with puberty is acne, or pimples. Acne is triggered by puberty hormones. Pimples usually start around the beginning of puberty and can stick around during adolescence (the teen years). You may notice pimples on your face, your upper back, or your upper chest. It helps to keep your skin clean, and your doctor will be able to offer some suggestions for clearing up acne. The good news about acne is that it usually gets better or disappears by the end of adolescence.

Putting The P.U. In Puberty

A lot of teens notice that they have a new smell under their arms and elsewhere on their bodies when they enter puberty, and it's not a pretty one.

That smell is body odor, and everyone gets it. As you enter puberty, the puberty hormones affect glands in your skin, and the glands make chemicals that smell bad. These chemicals put the scent in adolescent.

So what can you do to feel less stinky? Well, keeping clean is a good way to lessen the smell. You might want to take a shower every day, either in the morning before school, or the night before. Using deodorant (or deodorant with antiperspirant) every day can help keep body odor in check, too.

There's More?

Guys and girls will also notice other body changes as they enter puberty, and they're all normal changes. Girls might see and feel a white, mucous-like discharge from the vagina. This doesn't mean anything is wrong—it is just another sign of your changing body and hormones.

Guys will begin to get erections (this is when the penis fills with blood and becomes hard) sometimes. Erections happen when guys fantasize and think about sexual things or sometimes for no reason at all. They may experience something called nocturnal emissions (or wet dreams). This is when the penis becomes erect while a guy is sleeping, and he ejaculates. When a guy ejaculates, semen comes out of the penis—semen is a fluid that contains sperm. That's why they're called wet dreams—they happen when you're sleeping, and your underwear or the bed might be a little wet when you wake up. Wet dreams become less frequent as guys progress through puberty, and they eventually stop. Guys will also notice that their voices may "crack" and eventually get deeper.

Change Can Feel Kind Of Strange

Just as those hormones create changes in the way your body looks on the outside, they also create changes on the inside. While your body is adjusting to all the new hormones, so is your mind. During puberty, you might feel confused or have strong emotions that you've never experienced before. You may feel anxious about how your changing body looks.

You might feel overly sensitive or become easily upset. Some teens lose their tempers more than usual and get angry at their friends or families.

Sometimes it can be difficult to deal with all of these new emotions. Usually people aren't trying to hurt your feelings or upset you on purpose. It might not be your family or friends making you angry—it might be your new "puberty brain" trying to adjust. And while the adjustment can feel difficult in the beginning, it will gradually become easier. It can help to talk to someone and share the burden of how you're feeling—a friend or, even better, a parent, older sibling, or adult who's gone through it all before.

✎ What's It Mean?

Estrogen: A female hormone produced by the ovaries. Estrogen plays important roles in puberty, the menstrual cycle, and in reproduction. [1]

Follicle-Stimulating Hormone (FSH): A hormone secreted from the pituitary gland. In women, it stimulates the ovaries to develop eggs and to produce estrogen. In men, it stimulates the production of testosterone and sperm. [2]

Gonadotropin-Releasing Hormone (GnRH): A hormone made by the hypothalamus (part of the brain). GnRH causes the pituitary gland to make luteinizing hormone (LH) and follicle stimulating hormone (FSH). These hormones are involved in reproduction. [3]

Luteinizing Hormone (LH): A hormone that stimulates the production of sex hormones in men and women. [3]

Pituitary Gland: The pituitary gland is a small gland attached to the brain as part of the endocrine system. A gland is a group of cells that makes and then releases special chemicals called hormones. The pituitary gland makes different hormones that affect how other glands in the system release their hormones. Among other hormones, the pituitary makes growth hormone and endorphins, special chemicals that help provide natural pain relief from within the body. [1]

Testosterone: A hormone made mostly by the testes. This hormone causes many of the changes males deal with during puberty—deeper voices, body and facial hair, and the making of sperm. [1]

Source: [1] "Girlshealth.gov Web Site Glossary," The National Women's Health Information Center (NWHIC), U.S. Department of Health and Human Services, Office on Women's Health, December 2006. [2] Editor. [3] "Dictionary of Cancer Terms," National Cancer Institute, U.S. National Institutes of Health; cited July 2007.

You might have new, confusing feelings about sex—and a lot of questions. The adult hormones estrogen and testosterone are signals that your body is giving you new responsibilities, like the ability to create a child. That's why it's important to get all your questions answered.

It's easy to feel embarrassed or anxious when talking about sex, but you need to be sure you have all the right information. Some teens can talk to their parents about sex and get all their questions answered. But if you feel funny talking to your parents about sex, there are many other people to talk to, like your doctor, a school nurse, a teacher, a school counselor, or another adult you feel comfortable talking with.

Developing Differently

People are all a little different from one another, so it makes sense that they don't all develop in the same way. No two people are at exactly the same stage as they go through puberty, and everyone changes at his or her own pace. Some of your friends may be getting curves, whereas you don't have any yet. Maybe your best friend's voice has changed, and you think you still sound like a kid with a high, squeaky voice. Or maybe you're sick of being the tallest girl in your class or the only boy who has to shave.

But eventually everyone catches up, and the differences between you and your friends will even out. It's also good to keep in mind that there is no right or wrong way to look. That's what makes us human—we all have qualities that make us unique, on the inside and the outside.

Chapter 4

What Happens To Girls At Puberty?

Puberty

During adolescence, your body is going through many changes that are happening at a fast pace. While these changes might make you feel unsure of yourself at times, they can also be exciting. You are becoming a young woman. Learning about what is going on with your body will help you get through these changes.

What Is Puberty?

This time in your life when your body is changing is called puberty. For girls, puberty usually starts between the ages of 9 and 16. Sometimes, it can start as early as 6 or 7. Puberty for boys usually starts between the ages of 13 and 15, but may start as early as age 9. For both girls and boys, puberty takes several years. Major body changes have taken place for most girls, but not all, by the time they are 14. For boys, these changes happen at age 15 or 16.

How Do I Know If I'm In Puberty?

The first sign of puberty for most girls is growing breasts. Other changes include the following:

About This Chapter: Information in this chapter is from "Puberty," "Your Growth Spurt," "Body Hair," "Changes to Your Shape," "Changes to Your Breast," and "Changes to Your Mind," GirlsHealth.gov, sponsored by the National Women's Health Information Center, U.S. Department of Health and Human Services, February 2007.

- new body hair
- different body shape
- getting your period

Your Growth Spurt

During puberty, you will go through a growth spurt between ages 9 and 13. You will grow at a much faster pace than you had been growing. This growth process happens later for boys (between 10 and 16 years old), which is why you may find yourself taller than the boys in your class for a while.

Body Hair

Even before you get your first period, you will likely see new hair growing in your pubic area, under your arms, and on your legs. It will start out light and sparse, and then grow darker, coarser, and thicker as you go through puberty.

Although body hair is normal, some American women and girls remove the hair from their legs and underarms.

Changes To Your Shape

During puberty, you will not only get taller, you will also see other changes in your body such as wider hips, thighs, and bottom. Your body, which has both muscle and fat, will also start to have more fat compared to muscle than it did before. This is normal and you should not be too concerned.

These changes in your body might make you uncomfortable because it is so different than what you are used to. You also might think you look strange, or feel shy about your body around other people. Many people feel self-conscious during this phase, but remember that everyone goes through it. It is really common to struggle with body image (how you feel about your body), especially when there are many pictures of girls and women on television and in magazines with "perfect" bodies. Seeing these pictures may make you think there is something wrong with you if you are not as thin, but that is not true. Women and girls come in all shapes and sizes.

The size of your body does not have anything to do with your value as a person. It is important to have a healthy weight by having good eating habits and exercising regularly.

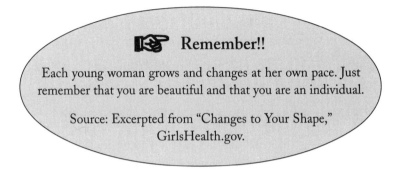

☞ Remember!!

Each young woman grows and changes at her own pace. Just remember that you are beautiful and that you are an individual.

Source: Excerpted from "Changes to Your Shape," GirlsHealth.gov.

Eating Disorders

Sometimes, worries about your body can become all you think about. Such thoughts may be part of an eating disorder. Eating disorders are serious health problems. Two of the most common eating disorders are anorexia nervosa and bulimia nervosa. Anorexia nervosa (often called anorexia) involves starving yourself and extreme weight loss. Bulimia nervosa (often called bulimia) involves binge eating (eating a lot of food at once) and then getting rid of the food by throwing up, using a laxative (which makes you go to the bathroom), or doing too much exercise.

Changes To Your Breasts

Having breasts is such a new thing for teen girls. When you start developing breasts, it is common to spend a lot of time thinking about how you look and how you compare to others. You may wish your breasts were bigger, or you may wish they were smaller. There may even be times when you cannot decide which you would prefer. The important thing to keep in mind is that every woman is different in the shape and size of her breasts. Your breasts do not need to look like your friend's breasts or a magazine model's breasts.

It is also important to know that it is very common for your two breasts to be different sizes, especially as you first start developing. Other people cannot tell that your breasts are different sizes. Also, exercises, vitamins, herbal teas, and creams, will not change the size of one or both of your breasts.

Throughout puberty, you might see or feel lumps and other changes in your breasts. During your period, they may even feel a little tender or sore. Most of the changes your breasts will go through are normal. To get used to these normal changes, you can do regular breast self-examinations (BSE). The best time to do it is about a week after your period starts. Let your doctor know if you find a lump or pain that you are not sure about, but keep in mind that harmless lumps are common in young women. Your doctor can show you exactly how to do a BSE.

Should I Wear A Bra? What About During Sports?

Having breasts is a normal part of being a woman, and you do not have to change your life because of them. If you find that exercise is not as comfortable, try wearing a sports bra with a snug fit for support.

Changes In Your Mind

During puberty, there are not just changes happening to your body, there are also changes taking place in your mind.

- You are able to understand more complex matters.

- You are starting to make your own moral choices.

- You know more about who you are and what your likes and dislikes are.

The teen years can seem like an emotional roller coaster, with worries about your changing body and the stress of school and social issues. While you might feel alone on this ride, it is important to know that everyone struggles with the highs and lows of adolescence.

Chapter 5

What Happens To Guys At Puberty?

A lot of changes happen as you grow up, especially as you reach puberty (say: pyoo-bur-tee), the name for the time when your body begins to develop and change. Girls start developing breasts and get their periods—signs they are growing into women. But how do boys know they are growing into men? Let's find out.

For a guy, there isn't just one event or sign that you're growing up. There are lots of them, including your body growing bigger, your voice changing, and hair sprouting everywhere. Most boys begin puberty between the ages of 10 and 15. But keep in mind that puberty starts when a boy's body is ready, and everyone grows at his own pace.

Here are some of the questions boys have.

Why Are Girls Taller Than Me?

You might have noticed that some of the girls you know are taller than the boys. But you've probably noticed that out of the adults you know, most of the men are taller than the women. What's going on?

About This Chapter: Information in this chapter is from "Boys and Puberty." This information was provided by KidsHealth, one of the largest resources online for medically reviewed health information written for parents, kids, and teens. For more articles like this one, visit www.KidsHealth.org, or www.TeensHealth.org. © 2005 The Nemours Foundation.

Well, girls get a head start on puberty—and growing taller—because they start these changes between the ages of 8 and 13. Most boys, on the other hand, don't begin until between the ages of 10 and 15. So that's why girls are often taller than boys during that time.

Many boys may catch up—and even grow taller than girls. But it's also important to remember that your genetics play a role in height. So if your mom and dad are tall, you're more likely to be tall. And if your mom and dad are kind of short, you may be short, too. But nothing is definite.

You have to wait and see how it turns out, but you can also talk to a doctor, if you're concerned. Remember—not every adult boy is tall. There are lots of men who are considered "short," but have gone on to have careers in the movies, the military, and even professional basketball.

When Will I Get Muscles?

During puberty, some boys might become worried about their bodies after seeing what some of their friends look like. For instance, lots of boys are concerned about their muscles. You may have already noticed some boys starting to get chest muscles (called the pectoralis muscles or pecs for short). Others may have broad shoulders (the deltoids, or delts for short). Other boys might still be slimmer and smaller.

> ♣ **It's A Fact!!**
> There aren't any exercises or magic pills to make you grow tall. But by being active and eating nutritious foods, you're helping your body grow up healthy, just the way it should.

Maybe you've considered lifting weights to help yourself get bigger. It's important to know that if you haven't quite reached puberty, this will tone your muscles, but it won't build up any muscles yet. Eating nutritious food and being active (like riding your bike, swimming, and playing sports) will help you be a kid who's strong and fit. In time, you'll reach puberty and you can start building your muscles, too.

If you decide to try lifting weights, first let your doctor know you are interested. He or she may tell you to hold off on weight lifting for a bit or give you some advice on how to start. If your doctor discourages weight lifting, there are some other ways to work out. Resistance bands, which are like big rubber bands, are a great way to help build your strength without putting too much strain on your muscles.

If your doctor recommends weight lifting, here are some tips:

- **Have a qualified coach or trainer supervise you.** It's smart to have somebody show you the proper way to lift weights. This will help you gain strength and prevent injury.

- **Use lighter weights.** Your coach or trainer can recommend the right amount. Lifting heavy weights can cause injuries and then you'll have to wait until you recover before you can work out again.

- **Do repetitions.** It's better to lift a smaller amount of weight a bunch of times than to try to lift a heavy weight once or twice.

- **Rest.** Let your body have a break at least every other day.

Do I Think About Girls Too Much Or Not Enough?

There is this girl who lives in your neighborhood, and you see her playing with her friends every afternoon when school is done. You get really hot, and your palms sweat when she says "hi" to you. That night you go to bed, and before you sleep, you have one last thought about her. Every day for the next few weeks you keep thinking about her. You might be wondering, "Why do I feel this way?" You just may have a crush.

Or perhaps your friend keeps talking about this one girl he thinks is so pretty. He goes on and on about how she tells funny jokes. He also tells you that he likes her. You think, "Why don't I feel or talk this way about a girl—am I supposed to?"

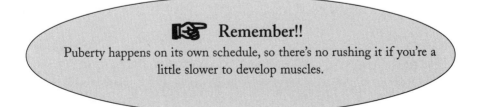

☞ Remember!!
Puberty happens on its own schedule, so there's no rushing it if you're a little slower to develop muscles.

Every boy has his own likes and dislikes. And during puberty, some boys are very friendly with girls, and others might be nervous about talking to girls. Thinking about someone you like is a normal process of puberty. And if you feel like you don't like any girls, that's fine, too. Eventually, you may find someone who makes you feel giddy inside. Only time will tell.

So why do you feel this way? The hormones in your body are becoming more active. As a result, you're starting to have more feelings. These feelings can confuse you and may leave you scared. This is natural because you are going through a new phase in your life.

Talking with a friend or an older person, like your brother or sister, may help you be less confused. Older people sometimes have more experience than you, so they can be good people to go to for advice.

What's Up With Body Hair?

Body hair really gets going during puberty. Some boys will start to notice hair growing on their face around the chin, on the cheeks, and above the lip. Also, hair grows on the chest, the armpits, and even down there in the pubic region. Remember that there's nothing to worry about because hair is just one of the body's many ways of telling you that you are entering adolescence.

You're growing hair in new places because hormones are telling your body that it is ready to change. One of these hormones is called testosterone, which is responsible for many of your body's changes. These hormones come from your pituitary (say: puh-too-uh-ter-ee) gland (a pea-shaped gland located at the bottom of your brain). The hormones travel through your bloodstream and tell different parts of your body to do stuff (like grow hair).

Boys don't really need to do anything about this new hair that's growing. Later, when you're a teen, and the hair gets thick enough on your face, you may want to talk with your parents about shaving.

Do I Smell?

You probably know what sweat is, but did you know that it's also called perspiration (say: pur-spuh-ray-shun)? How does it happen? Perspiration comes out of your skin, through tiny holes called pores, when your body gets hot.

Your body likes a temperature that is 98.6 degrees Fahrenheit (37 degrees Celsius). If you get hotter than that, your body doesn't like it, so then your body sweats. The sweat comes out of the skin, then evaporates (this means it turns from a liquid to a vapor) into the air, which cools you down. Sometimes this sweat, or wetness, can be smelly and create body odor (sometimes called BO). During puberty, your hormones are working all the time, which explains why you sweat a lot and, well, sometimes smell.

What makes it smelly? The sweat is made almost completely of water, with tiny amounts of other chemicals like ammonia (say: uh-mow-nyuh), urea (say: yoo-ree-uh), salts, and sugar. (Ammonia and urea are left over when your body breaks down protein.) Sweat by itself is not really smelly, but when it comes in contact with the bacteria on your skin (which everyone has) it becomes smelly.

But how can you keep yourself from being all sweaty and smelly? First, you can shower or bathe regularly, especially after playing sports or sweating a lot, like on a hot day. You can also use deodorant under your arms.

Deodorant comes in many good-smelling scents, or you can use one that's unscented. Some deodorants come in a white stick that you can twist up.

Lots of people put this on after showering or bathing before they put their clothes on. Otherwise, the white stick deodorants can leave white marks on your clothes. You can also choose a deodorant that's clear instead of white.

You can decide to wear a deodorant (which helps stop the smell) or a deodorant/antiperspirant (which helps stop the smell and the sweat). If you find these products aren't working for you, talk with your doctor.

What About Erections?

An erection is what happens when your penis hardens and fills up with blood. The penis will become bigger and stand out from the body. Boys will start to notice them occurring more often when they reach puberty. And they're perfectly normal.

An erection can happen even when you're sleeping. Sometimes you might wake up, and your underwear or bed is wet. You may worry that this means you wet your bed like when you were little, but chances are you had a nocturnal emission, or "wet dream." A wet dream is when semen (the fluid containing sperm) is discharged from the penis while a boy is asleep. Semen is released through the urethra—the same tube that urine (pee) comes out of. This is called ejaculation.

> **♣ It's A Fact!!**
> An erection can happen at any time. You can get many in one day or none at all. It depends on your age, sexual maturity, level of activity, and even the amount of sleep you get.

Wet dreams occur when a boy's body starts making more testosterone. This change for boys is a little bit like when a girl gets her period. It's a sign a boy is growing up and the body is preparing for the day in the future when a boy might decide to be a father. Semen contains sperm, which can fertilize a woman's egg and begin the process that ends with a baby being born.

Although some boys may feel embarrassed, or even guilty about having wet dreams, a boy can't help it. Almost all boys normally experience them at some time during puberty and even as adults.

But if you ever have pain or a problem with your penis or testicles, it is important that someone take you to the doctor. Maybe you've injured that area, or you find you have pain during an erection.

You may think, "Man, I don't want to go to the doctor for that!" But it's best to get problems like this checked out—and your doctor won't be embarrassed at all. It's a doctor's job to help you take care of your body—even that part.

Chapter 6

When Puberty Starts Early

What is precocious puberty (early puberty)?

Abnormally early puberty is called precocious puberty and is characterized by the early development of sexual characteristics in girls before the age of eight and in boys before the age of nine. Most children with the disorder grow fast at first, but also finish growing before reaching their full genetic height potential. Left untreated, most boys will not grow taller than 5 feet 2 inches and girls often do not grow taller than 5 feet.

What causes precocious puberty?

Early puberty and sexual development may be caused by tumors or growths of the ovaries, adrenal glands, pituitary gland, or brain. Other causes may include central nervous system abnormalities, family history of the disease, or certain rare genetic syndromes. In many cases, no cause can be found for the disorder. Two types of precocious puberty include the following:

- **Gonadotropin-Dependent Precocious Puberty:** Also known as central precocious puberty, this form of precocious puberty is the most

About This Chapter: "Precocious Puberty (Early Puberty)," is reprinted with permission from the Cincinnati Children's Hospital Medical Center website, http://www.cincinnatichildrens.org. © 2007 Cincinnati Children's Hospital Medical Center. All rights reserved.

common, affecting most girls with the disorder and half of boys with the disorder. The puberty is triggered by the premature secretion of gonadotropins (hormones responsible for puberty).

Researchers believe that the premature maturation of the hypothalamus-pituitary-ovaries axis causes this disorder in girls. However, in the majority of cases, no cause for the early secretion of gonadotropin hormones can be found.

- **Gonadotropin-Independent Precocious Puberty:** This is a form of precocious puberty that is not triggered by the early release of gonadotropin hormones.

What are the symptoms of precocious puberty?

The following are the most common symptoms of precocious puberty. However, each child may experience symptoms differently. As in normal puberty, symptoms of precocious puberty include the onset of secondary sexual characteristics, including the following:

- Girls:

  - breasts

  - pubic and underarm hair

  - menstruation

  - ovulation

- Boys:

  - enlarging penis and testicles

  - pubic and underarm hair

  - facial hair

  - spontaneous erections

  - production of sperm

  - development of acne

  - deepening of the voice

Other characteristics of the disorder include the following:

- typical moodiness associated with the hormonal changes

- increased aggression

- taller than peers, at first

How is precocious puberty diagnosed?

In addition to a complete medical history and physical examination, diagnosis of precocious puberty may include the following:

- x-ray—a diagnostic test, which uses invisible electromagnetic energy beams to produce images of internal tissues, bones, and organs onto film. A bone x-ray may be performed to determine bone age.

- measurement of gonadotropins (LH and FSH), estradiol, testosterone, and/or thyroid hormones

- ultrasound (also called sonography) of the adrenal glands and gonads (ovaries and testes)—a diagnostic imaging technique which uses high-frequency sound waves and a computer to create images of blood vessels, tissues, and organs. Ultrasounds are used to view internal organs as they function and to assess blood flow through various vessels.

- gonadotropin-stimulating hormone (GnRH) stimulation test (produced by the hypothalamus to stimulate the pituitary gland to release gonadotropins, which, in turn, stimulate the production of sex hormones in the gonads) to determine the form of precocious puberty (gonadotropin-dependent or gonadotropin-independent)

- magnetic resonance imaging (MRI)—a diagnostic procedure that uses a combination of large magnets, radio frequencies, and a computer to produce detailed images of organs and structures within the body.

What is the treatment for precocious puberty?

Specific treatment for precocious puberty will be determined by your physician based on the following:

- age, overall health, and medical history

- extent of the condition

- your tolerance for specific medications, procedures, or therapies

- expectations for the course of the condition

- your opinion or preference

The goal of treatment for precocious puberty is to stop, and possibly reverse, the onset of early puberty symptoms. Treatment will also depend on the type of precocious puberty and the underlying cause, if known.

♣ It's A Fact!!
New developments in hormone treatments for precocious puberty have led to the successful use of synthetic luteinizing-releasing hormone (LHRH). This synthetic hormone stops the sexual maturation process brought on by the disorder by halting the pituitary gland from releasing the gonadotropin hormones.

What is the emotional effect of precocious puberty?

Early puberty will cause a child's body to change much sooner than his/her peers. This sense of being different, coupled with the hormonal change-induced emotional mood swings, may make a child feel self-conscious. The child may feel uncomfortable about his/her sexual changes as well.

Chapter 7

When Puberty Starts Late

Jeff hates gym class. It's not that he minds playing soccer or basketball or any of the other activities. But he does dread going into the locker room at the end of class and showering in front of his friends. Although the other guys' bodies are growing and changing, his body seems to be stuck at a younger age. He's shorter than most of the other guys in his grade, and his voice hasn't deepened at all. It's embarrassing to still look like a little kid.

Abby knows what it's like to feel different, too. The bikini tops that her friends fill out lie flat on her. Most of them have their periods, too, and she hasn't had even a sign of one. Abby doesn't even really have to shave her legs or underarms, although she does it just to be like everyone else.

Both Jeff and Abby wonder and worry, "What's wrong with me?"

What Is Delayed Puberty?

Puberty is the time when your body grows from a child's to an adult's. You'll know that you are going through puberty by the way that your body changes. If you're a girl, you'll notice that your breasts develop and your pubic hair grows, that you have a growth spurt, and that you get your period

About This Chapter: Information in this chapter is from "Delayed Puberty." This information was provided by TeensHealth, one of the largest resources online for medically reviewed health information written for parents, kids, and teens. For more articles like this one, visit www.TeensHealth.org, or www.KidsHealth.org. © 2005 The Nemours Foundation.

(menstruation). The overall shape of your body will probably change, too—your hips will widen, and your body will become curvier.

If you're a guy, you'll start growing pubic and facial hair, have a growth spurt, and your testicles and penis will get larger. Your body shape will also begin to change—your shoulders will widen, and your body will become more muscular.

These changes are caused by the sex hormones (testosterone in guys and estrogen in girls) that your body begins producing in much larger amounts than before.

Puberty takes place over a number of years, and the age at which it starts and ends varies widely. It generally begins somewhere between the ages of 7 and 13 for girls, and somewhere between the ages of 9 and 15 for guys, although it can be earlier or later for some people. This wide range in age is normal, and it's why you may develop several years earlier (or later) than most of your friends.

Sometimes, though, people pass this normal age range for puberty without showing any signs of body changes. This is called delayed puberty.

What Causes Delayed Puberty?

There are several reasons why puberty may be delayed. Most often, it's simply a pattern of growth and development in a family. A guy or girl may find that his or her parent, uncle, aunt, brothers, sisters, or cousins developed later than usual, too. This is called constitutional delay (or being a late bloomer), and it usually doesn't require any kind of treatment. These teens will eventually develop normally, just later than most of their peers.

Medical problems also can cause delays in puberty. Some people with chronic illnesses like diabetes, cystic fibrosis, kidney disease, or even asthma may go through puberty at an older age because their illnesses can make it harder for their bodies to grow and develop. Proper treatment and better control of many of these conditions can help make delayed puberty less likely to occur.

A person who's malnourished—without enough food to eat or without the proper nutrients—may also develop later than peers who eat a healthy, balanced diet. For example, teens with the eating disorder anorexia nervosa often lose so much weight that their bodies can't develop properly. Girls who are extremely active in sports may be late developers because their level of exercise keeps them so lean. Girls' bodies require a certain amount of fat before they can go through puberty or get their periods.

Delayed puberty can also happen because of problems in the pituitary or thyroid glands. These glands produce hormones important for body growth and development.

Some people who don't go through puberty at the normal time have problems with their chromosomes (pronounced: kro-muh-soamz), which are made up of DNA that contain our body's construction plans. Problems with the chromosomes can interfere with normal growth processes.

Turner syndrome is an example of a chromosome disorder. It happens when one of a female's two X chromosomes is abnormal or missing. This causes problems with how a girl grows and with the development of her ovaries and

---

✎ What's It Mean?

Endocrinologist: A doctor who specializes in diagnosing and treating hormone disorders. [1]

Klinefelter Syndrome: A chromosomal condition that affects male sexual development. Most males with Klinefelter syndrome have one extra copy of the X chromosome in each cell. Because their testicles do not develop normally, affected males may have low levels of the hormone testosterone beginning during puberty. A lack of this hormone can lead to breast development (gynecomastia), reduced facial and body hair, and an inability to father children (infertility). [2]

Turner Syndrome: A chromosomal condition that affects development in females. Women with this condition tend to be shorter than average and are usually unable to conceive a child (infertile) because of an absence of ovarian function. [3]

Source: [1] "Dictionary of Cancer Terms," National Cancer Institute, U.S. National Institutes of Health; cited April 2007. [2] "Klinefelter syndrome," Genetics Home Reference, A Service of the U.S. National Library of Medicine, January 2006. [3] "Turner syndrome," Genetics Home Reference, A Service of the U.S. National Library of Medicine, September 2005.

production of sex hormones. Women who have untreated Turner syndrome are shorter than normal, are infertile, and may have other medical problems.

Males with Klinefelter syndrome are born with an extra X chromosome (XXY instead of XY). This condition can slow sexual development.

What Do Doctors Do?

The good news is that if there is a problem, doctors usually can help teens with delayed puberty to develop more normally. So if you are worried that you're not developing as you should, you should ask your parents to make an appointment with your doctor.

In addition to doing a physical examination, the doctor will take your medical history by asking you about any concerns and symptoms you have, your past health, your family's health, any medications you're taking, any allergies you may have, and other issues like growth patterns of your family members. He or she will chart your growth to see if your growth pattern points to a problem and also may order blood tests to check for thyroid, pituitary, chromosomal, or other problems. You may also have a "bone age" X-ray, which allows the doctor to see whether your bones are maturing normally.

In many cases, the doctor will be able to reassure you that there's no underlying physical problem; you're just a bit later than average in developing. If the doctor does find a problem, though, he or she might refer you to a pediatric endocrinologist (pronounced: en-doh-krih-nah-leh-jist), a

♣ It's A Fact!!
Some teens who are late developers may have a difficult time waiting for the changes of puberty to finally get going—even after a doctor has reassured them that they are normal. In some cases, doctors may offer teens a short course (usually a few months) of treatment with hormone medications to get the changes of puberty started. Usually, when the treatment is stopped a few months later, the teen's own hormones will take over from there to complete the process of puberty.

Source: © 2005 The Nemours Foundation

doctor who specializes in treating kids and teens who have growth problems, or to another specialist for further tests or treatment.

Dealing With Delayed Puberty

It can be really hard to watch your friends grow and develop when the same thing's not happening to you. You may feel like you're never going to catch up. People at school may joke about your small size or your flat chest. Even when the doctor or your parents reassure you that things will be OK eventually—and even when you believe they're right—it's difficult to wait for something that can affect how you feel about yourself.

If you're feeling depressed or having school or other problems related to delays in your growth and development, talk to your mom or dad, your doctor, or another trusted adult about finding a counselor or therapist you can talk to. This person can help you sort out your feelings and suggest ways to cope with them.

Delayed puberty can be difficult for anyone to accept and deal with—but it's a problem that usually gets solved. Ask for help if you have any concerns about your development. And remember that in most cases you will eventually catch up with your peers.

Chapter 8

Surviving Puberty: Moods And Emotions

You've probably noticed how your body changes during puberty. If you're a girl, your breasts get bigger and your hips widen. If you're a guy, your testicles and penis grow and your voice changes. Both girls and guys get hair under their arms and in their pubic regions, and they tend to sweat more and get acne.

Puberty also involves other developments that aren't as visible—changes in your emotions, moods, and thoughts. All these changes happen when your maturing brain and sex organs send hormones to the rest of your body, starting the process that helps you grow from a kid into an adult.

A New You

Many people who look back on their teen years describe them as a roller coaster of changing feelings. "You begin to have extremely powerful urges and feelings that you've never had before and have no experience dealing with," explains Dr. Jim Greer, a child and adolescent psychiatrist.

During puberty, you'll start to have more sexual thoughts and urges. You'll develop an attraction to girls or guys, and you may discover what having a crush on someone feels like.

About This Chapter: "Surviving Puberty: Moods and Emotions," reprinted with permission from Planned Parenthood® Federation of America, Inc. © 2007 PPFA. All rights reserved. For additional information, visit www.plannedparenthood.org.

As you get older, you begin to be able to think ahead, think about the past, and even analyze situations in a new way. Your new abilities allow you to have more complex thoughts and feelings, but one downside is that it can be harder to move on from negative emotions.

You may start to feel things more intensely. Life can be as dramatic as a juicy episode of The O.C.—one minute you may feel on top of the world, and the next minute you may feel pretty down in the dumps.

Tanya, 14, says she often worries about her looks and what guys think of her. "I can feel fine about myself, and then one wrong look from the guy I like makes me want to freak," she says.

While all these changes can be exciting, they can also be a source of stress for teens. So how can you deal with your changing body and moods?

Talk About It

One good place to start is to talk to your parents or another trusted adult. "It's common for teenagers to feel uncomfortable and embarrassed exploring these perfectly normal, healthy, and necessary emotions," says Dr. Greer. But puberty is nothing to be embarrassed about. Your parents have been through it—they can let you know what to expect and give you tips on how to deal with changes. Older sisters, brothers, or cousins can be helpful, too.

☞ Remember!!
It's Perfectly Normal

Although your feelings may seem out of control, try to remember that your changing moods are a normal part of growing up. And by reminding yourself that it's okay to feel the way you do, and that you don't have to act on your feelings, you can feel more confident and in control as you begin to get to know the exciting "new you."

Let It All Out

Many teens find that writing, acting, music, and art are good ways to manage stress and help them feel more in control of their moods. Your changing hormones may leave you hyper and restless, and finding a creative outlet—or doing something physical, like dancing or playing sports—can be a great way to release excess energy.

And speaking of excess energy—some teens find that they are sexually aroused a lot when they are going through puberty. While being aroused a lot can feel embarrassing or out of control, rest assured that it is normal. As you get older and get more used to arousal, it will seem less intrusive and more in control. Some teens choose to masturbate to release sexual feelings and others just wait for the feelings to pass.

Part Two

Protecting Your Sexual Health

Chapter 9

Seven Steps To Sexual Health

Maybe this year you've resolved to get better grades, stop fighting with your siblings, or save up your allowance. These are all great New Year's resolutions, but how about adding one more to the mix that'll improve your body, your mind—and your sex life? This year, think about how you can be sexually healthy.

Here are seven things you can do to improve your sexual health:

1. Get the facts.

Gather the information you need to make healthy sexual decisions—facts about anatomy, birth control, sexually transmitted infections, and safer sex. There is a lot of misinformation out there, so be sure to check your facts against trusted sources.

2. Get perspective.

Forget expectations about how you "should" feel or look or express your sexuality. Listen instead to what your body and mind are telling you. Our bodies have a great capacity for pleasure—whether or not we look like a perfect "10"—and there is a far greater variety of sexual expression than what's depicted in mainstream media.

About This Chapter: "Seven Steps to Sexual Health," reprinted with permission from Planned Parenthood® Federation of America, Inc. © 2007 PPFA. All rights reserved. For additional information, visit www.plannedparenthood.org.

3. Know thyself.

Facts alone can't improve your sexual health. Sexual health is rooted in self-awareness and self-knowledge—and you can't find that information in a book or online.

A key component of sexual health is knowing your body—what it looks like, how it works, and how it feels. Becoming more familiar with your sexual anatomy can help reduce the sense of shame or mystery some people have about their sex organs. People who are familiar with their sex organs are more likely to detect a possible infection or other health problem. And exploring through masturbation—touching one's own sex organs for pleasure—is one of the primary ways people learn what they do and do not enjoy sexually.

> ## ♣ It's A Fact!!
> Sexual health is something that affects all of us, whether we're currently sexually active or not. Sexual health is about more than using birth control, practicing safer sex, or being free of infection or dysfunction. It's about being emotionally, physically, and mentally aware of what you want and need sexually. It's also about communication and responsibility.

This kind of self-awareness informs relationships as well. You can begin to ask yourself bigger questions: What kinds of sex play do you want to engage in, and what kinds would you rather not? Are you attracted to women or men or both? How can you pursue your pleasure safely?

The better you know yourself, the better you are able to share yourself with another person.

4. Communicate.

Communication is a vital part of any healthy sexual relationship.

When becoming sexual with a new partner, it's important to talk about expectations. What do you want from a sexual relationship—physically and emotionally? What are your boundaries? Communicating these expectations helps to put everyone on the same page.

It's also important to discuss birth control and safer sex. Which risks are you willing to take—and which ones aren't you willing to take? How will you and your partner share both the pleasure and the responsibility of a sexual relationship?

5. Get a check-up.

Maintaining your sexual health is not something you accomplish all on your own. A health care provider can be a great ally.

Whether or not you are sexually active, it's important to take proper care of your reproductive and sexual health. For women, this means getting regular pelvic and breast exams. For men, this means getting your prostate and testicles checked. Depending on the risks you've taken, you may want to be tested for sexually transmitted infections. You and your health care provider can decide together which tests may be right for you.

6. Get support.

One obstacle to sexual health is sexual abuse. The World Health Organization estimates that as many as one in four women and one in ten men have been the victims of some form of sexual abuse, including rape. Many find support groups or individual therapy to be helpful. Support groups and individual therapy can provide a place where fears and concerns can be safely expressed and explored.

Substance abuse and mental health issues such as depression, eating disorders, or anxiety can also affect your sexual health. Getting support in dealing with these issues can help ensure that you are making healthy choices when it comes to your sex life.

7. Enjoy yourself.

Enjoying our sexuality is a normal, natural part of life. For many people, however, there is so much guilt, embarrassment, and shame associated with sex that the pleasure is lost. A social climate that demonizes sex doesn't help.

It's important to our sexual health to be able to enjoy our sexuality and the way we express ourselves sexually. The first six steps to sexual health can help us become more responsible and secure in our sexuality and in our sexual relationships. They provide a foundation for allowing us to enjoy our sexual selves to the fullest.

Chapter 10

Finding The Right Clinic And The Services They Offer

Why Visit The Clinic?

You don't have to be pregnant or have an infection to go to the clinic.

Going now can help protect you in the future.

Where To Go

Depending on where you live and what your money situation and insurance are like, you have lots of different options:

- Teen clinic

- Private doctor

- Free clinic

- Hospital clinic

- Health department

- Private clinic (like Planned Parenthood)

Call Around

- Look for sliding-scale fees (discounts).

- Ask if appointments are necessary.

- Ask about after school and weekend hours.

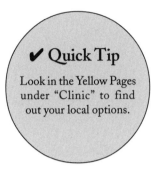

✔ Quick Tip

Look in the Yellow Pages under "Clinic" to find out your local options.

The Scene

"My friend said that the clinic was unpleasant, but my experience was different. I talked with a counselor and I learned a lot."

Every clinic is different. Find out what services are available before you go. If you have a long wait, you can read or hang out with other patients.

Be Prepared

It helps to bring a friend. Don't let them rush you. If you don't understand something, ask and ask again.

Birth Control Counseling

"My boyfriend and I have decided to have sex, and we want to use protection. I came to the clinic to get counseling on birth control and sexually transmitted infections (STIs)."

When you go to the clinic for birth control counseling, make sure you learn about all of your options—not just the ones you've heard of. Keep your mind open to the possibilities.

For some methods, you need a pelvic exam and/or a prescription.

Pregnancy Test

"I'm really scared about this test. I wish we had used protection."

"I feel much better with him here. What will we do if I'm pregnant?"

What's a pregnancy test like? You pee in a cup or take a blood test. Get your results (at the same visit) and talk with a counselor.

If you're not pregnant, be sure to get information on birth control so that you can protect yourself.

If you are pregnant, be sure to take the time to talk about your options—adoption, abortion, keeping the baby. (One out of every six pregnancies ends in miscarriage.)

Ask about emergency conceptive pills, which can be taken within 120 hours (five days) after unprotected sex to prevent pregnancy.

Clinics Are For You Too, Guys

You can go for STI testing (sexually transmitted infections), testicular exam and checkup, birth control counseling with your girlfriend, and free condoms. Don't be afraid to ask questions.

"I woke up this morning and my penis was all itchy and burning, and there was stuff coming out of it. My friends say I might have an infection since I didn't use a condom. He told me to get it checked out at the clinic."

You don't have to have an infection to go to the clinic. It's a good idea to get regular checkups.

Testicular Exam: Taking Care Of Yourself

When you go to the clinic for a regular checkup, or if you think you have a sexually transmitted infection (STI), the doctor will examine your penis and testicles (balls) for lumps, sores, and discharge. (Yea, we know, this is kind of uncomfortable.)

They might also get blood and urine samples to check for STIs. You can examine yourself at home every month to look for changes. Ask the doctor for more information.

The Pelvic Exam

Don't let friends' stories scare you. Pelvic exams are a great way to learn more about your body.

What really happens? First, the doctor looks at your vulva (labia, ure-thra, clitoris, vagina). Next, the doctor inserts the bills of the speculum into your vagina and opens it to see your cervix. Finally, the bimanual exam—the doctor puts one finger in your vagina and presses down on your abdomen with the other hand to locate your uterus and ovaries.

You need to have a pelvic exam once a year after age 18 or once you start having sex. Don't delay.

Positive Tips For Your Pelvic Exam

- Relax. Take a deep breath. If you're tense, it might be uncomfortable.

- Have the doctor show you the speculum and explain the exam.

- If you want to, sit up during the exam and ask for a mirror so that you can watch.

- Listen to your Walkman or daydream to help you relax.

- If you want, ask for the speculum after the exam so that you can become more familiar with that part of your body.

We know it can be uncomfortable, but if you relax it will be easier. Use this as a learning opportunity.

Breast Exams

"My doctor taught me how to examine my own breasts."

You can do it in the shower, in your room, or looking in the mirror.

Positive Tips

- Start now and make it a habit every month.

- The best time is right after your period.

- Put a reminder in your calendar.

If you find anything unusual, go to the clinic.

One of eight women will get breast cancer. Exams help you find it before it spreads.

Questions For The Clinic?

If possible, it's wise to go with your partner so that you can learn together and have support. When you go to the clinic, you deserve to get all the available information on your health and your options. Here are some good questions to keep in mind. It helps to write them down.

- How much will my visit cost?
- What is the best method of birth control for me?
- Can my partner come with me?
- Are you going to call my house with test results? (You can tell them not to.)
- How can I best protect myself from STIs?

It's Not Just A Clinic

We know that sometimes it is hard for teenagers to find someone they can trust to talk with about personal situations such as sexual orientation, family, rape, or alcohol or drug abuse.

Take advantage of your visit to the clinic to ask for help. Clinic staff can usually help you find a place in your community that can provide support. Just ask.

Chapter 11

Facts On American Teens' Sexual And Reproductive Health

Sexual Activity

- Nearly half (46%) of all 15–19-year-olds in the United States have had sex at least once.

- By age 15, only 13% of teens have ever had sex. However, by the time they reach age 19, 7 in 10 teens have engaged in sexual intercourse.

- Most young people have sex for the first time at about age 17, but do not marry until their middle or late 20s. This means that young adults are at risk of unwanted pregnancy and sexually transmitted infections (STIs) for nearly a decade.

- Teens are waiting longer to have sex than they did in the past. Some 13% of females and 15% of males aged 15–19 in 2002 had sex before age 15, compared with 19% and 21%, respectively, in 1995.

- The majority (59%) of sexually experienced teen females had a first sexual partner who was 1–3 years their senior. Only 8% had first partners who were 6 or more years older.

About This Chapter: Guttmacher Institute, "Facts on American Teens' Sexual and Reproductive Health," *In Brief*, New York: Guttmacher, 2006, http://www.guttmacher.org/pubs/fb_ATSRH.html, accessed April 2007.

- More than three-quarters of teen females report that their first sexual experience was with a steady boyfriend, a fiancé, a husband, or a cohabiting partner.

- Ten percent of young women aged 18–24 who had sex before age 20 reported that their first sex was involuntary. The younger they were at first intercourse, the higher the proportion.

- Twelve percent of teen males and 10% of teen females have had heterosexual oral sex but not vaginal intercourse.

- The proportion of teens who had ever had sex declined from 49% to 46% among females and from 55% to 46% among males between 1995 and 2002.

> ♣ It's A Fact!!
> Sex is rare among very young teens, but becomes more common in the later teenage years.

Contraceptive Use

- A sexually active teen who does not use contraceptives has a 90% chance of becoming pregnant within a year.

- The majority of sexually experienced teens (74% of females and 82% of males) used contraceptives the first time they had sex.

- The condom is the most common contraceptive method used at first intercourse; it was used by 66% of sexually experienced females and 71% of males.

- Nearly all sexually active females (98% in 2002) have used at least one method of birth control. The most common methods used are the condom (used at least once by 94%) and the pill (used at least once by 61%).

- Nearly one-quarter of teens who used contraceptives the last time they had sex combined two methods, primarily the condom and a hormonal method.

- At most recent sex, 83% of teen females and 91% of teen males used contraceptives. These proportions represent a marked improvement since 1995, when only 71% of teen females and 82% of teen males had used a contraceptive method at last sex.

Access To Contraceptive Services

- Twenty-one states and the District of Columbia explicitly allow all minors to consent to contraceptive services without a parent's involvement. Two states (Texas and Utah) require parental consent for contraceptive services in state-funded family planning programs.

- Ninety percent of publicly funded family planning clinics counsel clients younger than 18 about abstinence and the importance of communicating with parents about sex.

- Sixty percent of teens younger than 18 who use a clinic for sexual health services say their parents know they are there.

- Among those whose parents do not know, 70% would not use the clinic for prescription contraception if the law required that their parents be notified.

- One in five teens whose parents do not know they obtain contraceptive services would continue to have sex but would either rely on withdrawal or not use any contraceptives if the law required that their parents be notified of their visit.

- Only 1% of all minor adolescents who use sexual health services indicate that their only reaction to a law requiring their parents' involvement for prescription contraception would be to stop having sex.

- Of the 18.9 million new cases of STIs each year, 9.1 million (48%) occur among 15–24-year-olds.

- Although 15–24-year-olds represent only one-quarter of the sexually active population, they account for nearly half of all new STIs each year.

- Human papillomavirus (HPV) infections account for about half of STIs diagnosed among 15–24-year-olds each year. HPV is extremely common, often asymptomatic, and generally harmless. However, certain types, if left undetected and untreated, can lead to cervical cancer.

- In June 2006, the U.S. Food and Drug Administration approved the vaccine Gardasil as safe and effective for use among girls and women aged 9–26. The vaccine prevents infection with the types of HPV most likely to lead to cervical cancer.

- Half of new HIV infections (about 20,000) each year occur among youth aged 15–24.

Pregnancy

- Each year, almost 750,000 women aged 15–19 become pregnant. Overall, 75 pregnancies occur every year per 1,000 women aged 15–19; this rate has declined 36% since its peak in 1990.

- The majority of the decline in teen pregnancy rates is due to more consistent contraceptive use; the rest is due to higher proportions of teens choosing to delay sexual activity.

- Black women have the highest teen pregnancy rate (134 per 1,000 women aged 15–19), followed by Hispanics (131 per 1,000) and non-Hispanic whites (48 per 1,000).

- The pregnancy rate among black teens decreased 40% between 1990 and 2000, more than the overall U.S. teen pregnancy rate declined during the same period (36%).

- Eighty-two percent of teen pregnancies are unplanned; they account for about 1 in 5 of all unintended pregnancies annually.

- Two-thirds of all teen pregnancies occur among 18–19-year-olds.

- Teen pregnancy rates are much higher in the United States than in many other developed countries—twice as high as in England and Wales or Canada, and eight times as high as in the Netherlands or Japan.

Chapter 12

Talking With Your Parents About Sex

Let's Face It—Teens Have To Deal With Many Tough Issues

Teens have to deal with many tough issues including the following:

- Trying to do well in school

- Resisting peer pressure

- Making decisions about sex and sexuality

- Drinking alcohol or experimenting with drugs

- Trying to fit in

Some of these issues are related to your sexuality. Sexuality is an important part of who you are. Sexuality has to do with how you express yourself, how you feel about your body, the way you act in relationships, and how you interact with males and females. Facing sexuality issues can be hard.

The good news is, there are many people in your life who can help you sort out your feelings, answer your questions, and help you make good decisions. Your parents, family members, teachers, school counselors, and other trusted adults are all people who care about you and want to help.

About This Chapter: Information in this chapter is from "The Importance of Talking to Your Parents About Sex and Sexuality," © Planned Parenthood of New York City. Reprinted with permission; cited April 2007.

It can be a little scary to ask questions, but this chapter will help you feel more comfortable and confident about communicating with your parents and other important adults in your life about sexuality and growing up.

Getting Started

Some teens are afraid to approach their parents or other adults because they are afraid of negative reactions. Some fear that if they ask questions about sexuality their parents will assume that they are sexually active. But you would be surprised at how willing your parents and other adults in your lives are to talk about these issues. While parents and other adults may sometimes be uncomfortable talking about sexuality issues, they have your best interests at heart and want to help you.

One thing to do before you get started is to think about the questions you want to ask. You may even want to write them down so that you feel prepared and less anxious. Here are some questions that other teens have asked their parents:

- How are things different now than when you were growing up?

- What was it like for you growing up as a teen?

- When will my body begin changing?

- What do you think is the right age to begin dating?

- How do you feel about me going out alone on a date?

- How do you feel about me dating someone older/younger?

- How do you know when you are in love?

- What is the right age to engage in sexual activity?

- How do you feel about teens having sex?

These questions will also give you a sense of what your parents' and other adults' values are about dating, relationships, and sexuality.

Remember, many parents did not receive much sexuality education themselves, so talking about sexuality may be hard for them. They may appear uncomfortable at first, but they still want to talk to you. One way to begin is to ask your parents what their parents taught them about sexuality. That conversation can open up a lot of different topics and help you to understand your parents' point of view.

When Is The Right Time To Talk?

There are many everyday opportunities to talk to parents about sexuality issues. These "askable moments" include while watching a television show or movie; listening to the radio; reading a story, magazine, or newspaper; or just during everyday conversation.

Of course, you'll want to talk when adults are most receptive, so you may want to avoid times when your parents are talking on the telephone, entertaining guests, or feeling tired or upset. Let your parents know that you have important things to talk about, and ask them to set aside some time to talk with you.

While it may be hard to get started, once you do, you'll see that you and your parents will begin to build stronger relationships with better communication.

What If I Am Not Ready To Talk To My Parents?

Your parents are the best people to talk to about sexuality issues. If your parents are not available, you can also speak with other trusted adults—older siblings, family members, teachers, school counselors, and clergy, for example. There are also other places where you can get good information in an anonymous, safe way.

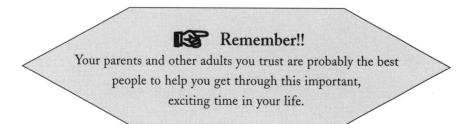

☞ **Remember!!**

Your parents and other adults you trust are probably the best
people to help you get through this important,
exciting time in your life.

Chapter 13

How Do You Know When You're Ready For Sex?

Am I Ready For Sex?

This is a question that almost everyone will ask themselves at some point in their lives, but unfortunately not many people will be able to answer it with a definite "yes" or "no."

Having sex for the first time can be complicated. It can lead to pregnancy, and if your partner has human immunodeficiency virus (HIV) or a sexually transmitted disease (STD) (and you might not always know they do), you can become infected too. There can also be emotional consequences to having sex with someone—it can really change a relationship, and not always for the better. Sex can be enjoyable with the right person, but it's very easy to make mistakes and end up hurt, which is why people advise you: "don't have sex until you're ready!"

About This Chapter: This chapter begins with "Am I ready for sex?" © 2007 AVERT (www.avert.org). All rights reserved. Reprinted with permission. Text under the heading "Virginity And The First Time" is from "SexSmarts Survey—Virginity and The First Time" (#3368), The Henry J. Kaiser Family Foundation, October 2003. This information was reprinted with permission from the Henry J. Kaiser Family Foundation. The Kaiser Family Foundation, based in Menlo Park, California, is a nonprofit, private operating foundation focusing on the major health care issues facing the nation and is not associated with Kaiser Permanente or Kaiser Industries. To view the complete text of this document, visit www.kff.org.

Of course it's all very well saying this, but how do you know when you're ready? Legally, you aren't allowed to have sex with anyone until you're over the age of consent. But it takes more than just legally being the right age to make you ready for sex—you need to be emotionally ready too.

We obviously don't know you, so you're the only person who can truly judge if you're ready to have sex. But we can suggest some questions that will hopefully help you to work it out.

Are you doing this because YOU want to?

Or are you thinking about doing it because someone else wants you to? Maybe you're not sure you're ready, but your partner is keen? Or perhaps there's a bit of "peer pressure"—all your friends seem to be doing it, so you feel you should be too?

Do any of the following sound familiar?

- "You would if you loved me!"
- "It's only natural!"
- "Everyone else is doing it!"
- "Don't you want to make our relationship stronger?"
- "You'll have to do it sometime—why not now, with me?"
- "I'll be gentle, and it'll be really great, I promise!"
- "I'll only put it in for a second."

If you're hearing things like this, then you should think carefully. These are not the right reasons to have sex. A partner who's saying things like this is trying to put pressure on you and doesn't really care whether you're ready or not—this person doesn't respect your feelings, and they're probably not the right person to have sex with.

Nor should you have sex just because your friends are saying things like the following:

- "You mean you've never done it?"
- "I lost it when I was twelve."

- "Yeah, I've had sex loads of times."

- "You're a virgin, you wouldn't understand."

- "No one will be interested in you if they hear you're frigid."

- "It's amazing—you don't know what you're missing!"

It may feel like your friends are all more experienced and knowledgeable, but we guarantee they're probably not. Many of them will only be saying things like this because they think everyone will laugh at them if they admit they've never really done anything. Besides, being sexually experienced at a young age doesn't necessarily make someone mature or sensible—in fact, it indicates the opposite.

Do I know my partner well enough?

If you've only just met your partner, haven't been going out with them very long, or perhaps don't even really know them, then sex is never going to be a really good experience because there won't be much trust between you. If you've never even kissed the person you're with, then you're definitely not ready to have sex with them.

Sex can leave you feeling very vulnerable afterwards in a way you might not be prepared for, so it's better to be with someone that you know is likely to be sticking around. Usually, you'll have better sex with someone you know really well, are comfortable with, and who you can talk to openly about relationships and feelings. Sex will be best with someone you love.

Is it legal?

The age of consent differs between countries. In most states of the U.S. for instance, it ranges between 16 and 18. In the United Kingdom, it's 16. And in India, it's 16. For additional information about age of consent, go to http://www.avert.org/teensex.htm.

So why do countries have a legal age for having sex? Because this is the age when the government believes young people are mature enough to handle the responsibilities that come with having sex. All too often people think they are ready when they're not. Age of consent laws are also designed to prevent older people from taking advantage of children and young teenagers who may not understand the consequences of having sex, or even what sex is.

Do I feel comfortable enough with my partner to do this, and to do it sober?

It's natural to feel a little embarrassed and awkward the first time you have sex with someone because it's not something you've ever done before. Your boyfriend or girlfriend will probably feel the same. But if you don't trust your partner enough not to laugh at you, or you don't feel you can tell them you've never had sex before, then it's far better to wait until you can.

And if you think you'll have to drink a lot of alcohol before you do it so you feel relaxed enough, or you only find yourself thinking about having sex when you're drunk, then that suggests you're not ready. A lot of people lose their virginity when they're drunk or on drugs, and then regret it. So if you're worried that you're going to be in a situation where you might be tempted to do something you wouldn't do normally, restrict your drinking, keep off the drugs, or make sure you stick with a sober friend who can look after you.

Do I know enough about sex?

Do you know what happens during sex? Do you know how it works, what it's for, and how and why a woman can get pregnant? Do you know about sexually transmitted infections? Lots of people worry that they're going to make a fool of themselves or do something wrong. Well, you shouldn't have to worry if you're with a partner who cares about you—he/she won't laugh. And if you're not with a partner who cares, you probably shouldn't be doing it. Physically, sex is actually quite simple, but the more you know, the more comfortable you'll feel. For more information, go to http://www.avert.org/yngindx.htm.

Will I be glad when I'm older that I lost my virginity at the age I am now?

Imagine that you're looking back at yourself in ten years time. What do you think you'll think then about how and when you lost your virginity? Is there any way in which you might regret it? The answer should be "no"—if it's not, you're probably not ready yet.

Can I talk to my partner about this easily?

If you can't talk about sex, then you're not ready to have sex. It's as simple as that. Being honest about how you're feeling will make it easier for both of you, and will make sex better in the future.

Do I know how to have sex safely?

It's really important that you know how to protect against pregnancy, sexually transmitted infections (STIs), and HIV. Again, this is something you need to talk to your boyfriend or girlfriend about before the event, so you're both okay about what you're going to use. For information on contraception options, go to http://www.avert.org/cpills.htm.

Especially with things like condoms, it's good to have a bit of practice putting them on and to feel okay about doing it. It's not enough just to get a condom if you're not confident enough to use it—they're no good if they stay in your pocket the whole time.

Do we both want to do this?

You may decide that you are ready, but it might be that your partner isn't, even if they have had sexual partners before. For sex to work, you both have to be willing to do it. Don't ever pressure anyone to have sex if they're not sure—this is very wrong, and it'll cost you your partner's respect and the respect of other people.

Also, there's a fine line between pressuring someone to have sex and forcing someone to have sex. If you put too much pressure on someone, it can become force—and if you force someone into sex, you can be prosecuted for rape.

Does sex fit in with my/their personal beliefs?

It may be that you, your partner, or your family have beliefs that say sex at a young age (or before marriage) is wrong. Do you feel comfortable going against these views? Will it cause you unnecessary worry and guilt if you do (or don't)? Some young people will have sex simply because their family has banned them from doing so, even if they don't realize that this is the reason. Having sex as an act of rebellion may feel great at the time, but

if anything goes wrong, you face a very difficult situation, as you may not be able to
rely on your family's support.

Even if everything goes well, keeping sex (and all the emotions that go
with it) a secret can be very hard—so,
if possible, you should make sure you
have someone else to talk to that you
can trust to keep it to themselves.

> 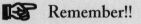 **Remember!!**
> The decision to have sex should
> be an agreement between you and
> your partner, and while other people
> may help or influence your decision,
> they shouldn't make it for you.
>
> Source: © 2007 AVERT
> (www.avert.org)

So, how did you do?

If you answered "yes" to all ten of these questions, then you're probably
pretty much ready, as long as both of you feel okay about it.

If you didn't, then there are probably some issues you need to work through
first, because all of these questions are important.

First time sex is always going to be scary whatever age you are when you
have it. It can sometimes seem like losing your virginity is the most important thing in the world.

Virginity And The First Time

When it comes to sex, for many teens the perception can be very different
from the reality. By almost equal measures, teens overestimate and underestimate the percentage of their peers who are sexually active. Some of these differing views may be related to how they define "sex" today, specifically whether they
consider oral sex to be sex or not. Teens are split when it comes to this issue.

> **Remember!!**
> You can't get your virginity back once it's gone, so what is
> really important is that you have enough respect for yourself to wait until
> you're truly ready and can truly trust the person you're with.
>
> Source: © 2007 AVERT (www.avert.org)

Whatever they think about who is having sex, the large majority of teens surveyed see value in waiting. Virtually all—including as many of those who are sexually active as those who are not—say being a virgin in high school is a "good thing" and that teens who choose not to have sex are "supported" in that decision. Teens also acknowledge that delaying sex has a variety of benefits including; respect, control, and freedom from worry about sexual health risks like pregnancy and sexually transmitted diseases (STDs).

The third of teens in this survey who have had sex also cite a variety of factors as affecting their decision, including feeling that the time was right, being in love, or having found the right person. However, less positive factors, such as peer pressure and drugs and alcohol, also played a role for some teens.

This survey snapshot explores perceptions of virginity and first sexual activity among adolescents. It is based on a national random sample telephone survey with 508 teens ages 15 to 17 conducted from June 4 to 9, 2003 by International Communications Research (ICR) for the Kaiser Family Foundation and *seventeen* magazine.

Everybody's Doing It…Right?

Wrong. According to the Centers for Disease Control and Prevention, about half of teens in high school have had sexual intercourse. Or looked at another way, half have not (CDC, Youth Risk Behavior Surveillance data 2001). While many teens have a generally accurate picture of teen sexuality today, some are off the mark. About a third of teens (34%) in this survey overestimate how many of their peers are sexually active, while another quarter (24%) underestimate this rate. And, few (3%) realize their generation is actually less likely to be sexually active than that from a decade ago (CDC, Youth Risk Behavior Surveillance data 1991–2001).

Contributing to these varied perceptions about sex may be that young people often have differing views about what constitutes sex. When it comes to defining virginity, teens are evenly divided on whether or not oral sex is "sex." Half say no (50%), half say yes (48%).

Virginity And Waiting

Teens overwhelmingly value virginity and waiting, regardless of their personal decision. More than nine in ten agree that being a virgin is a "good thing." A majority also say teens who choose to wait are "supported" in their decision. Still, many acknowledge that waiting to have sex can be a "difficult decision" nonetheless. While most agree that

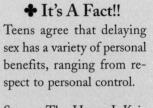

♣ It's A Fact!!
Teens agree that delaying sex has a variety of personal benefits, ranging from respect to personal control.

Source: The Henry J. Kaiser Family Foundation

gender doesn't make a difference, a little over a quarter say it is easier for girls than boys to stick to a decision not to be sexually active in high school.

Most teens agree that it is important to be a virgin in high school, but what about after graduation? Among teens who have not had sex, fewer than ten percent say they are waiting to have sex until they are out of school. More than four in ten are waiting for a committed relationship, and more than a third are waiting for marriage.

Why Wait?

So what are they waiting for? Generally, teens agree that monogamy and maturity are central to their decision-making. When asked what age it is appropriate to lose your virginity, teens most frequently said 18 or when you are married. Among teens surveyed who had not had sex, over three-fourths agreed that they were waiting to have sex when they are in a committed relationship or married.

More than nine in ten note that abstaining from sexual activity in high school results in having respect for yourself and enjoying the respect of your family. Waiting also leads teens to feel like they are in control of their relationships and are behaving consistently with their moral or religious beliefs. Lower on the list, but still significant, is respect from friends. General worry or concerns about sexual health risks were also considerable.

The First Time

Most adolescents surveyed agree that sexual activity is most appropriate among people aged 18 and older or those who are married or in committed relationships. Over a third agree that one should be at least 18 years old when you lose your virginity—and about a quarter believe you should wait for marriage. Very few—two percent of teens surveyed—consider sex under the age of 15 to be appropriate. Girls were more likely than boys surveyed to volunteer that marriage was when they personally felt it was best to lose your virginity. Among those who have already had sexual intercourse, almost half believe it is best to wait—until 18 or older (29%), or for marriage (17%)—in spite of their own decision.

Teens are divided in their views about what happens the "first time." While 41 percent believe in most instances it is "planned," more than half (57%) say often sex is just something that "happens." There is no significant difference in the views of teens who have already had sex as opposed to those who have not. Part of the reason so many teens may perceive the "first time" experience as unplanned may be the involvement of drugs or alcohol. Eight in ten have the impression that alcohol or drugs are a part of many teens' first sexual experience, and nearly one in five sexually active teens surveyed said that they were using drugs or alcohol when they lost their virginity.

Over a third (38%) of both sexually active teens and those who are not sexually active agree that when you lose your virginity you "just want to get it over with." These feelings of anxiety may contribute to many teens' belief that they don't have to worry about their sexual health or contraception the first time. Almost one fifth (17%) of teens surveyed agreed that you don't have to use birth control or condoms the first time you have sex, and over half (54%) say that you aren't even thinking about STDs, including HIV/AIDS. This is surprising considering that teens report that pregnancy, human immunodeficiency virus/acquired immune deficiency (HIV/AIDS), and other STDs are top concerns during their first sexual experience.

Decision-Making

Among the two thirds of teens in this survey who reported that they had not yet had sexual intercourse, many report being worried about pregnancy, HIV/AIDS and other STDs. What they have been taught at home and at school also influenced many of these young people's decision to wait, as well as their own personal values. About half cited a general lack of opportunity as a factor. Most sexually active teens indicated that their decision to have sex had to do with a sense of maturity and intimacy with a partner. Most felt "ready," like the time was "right" for them to lose their virginity, and they were with the "right person." Three fourths agreed that they had been with their partner "for a long time," and seven in ten were "in love." Over half

thought they would marry their first sexual partner. About two-thirds (65%) were in what they defined as a "serious relationship" when they first had sex, and most (83%) reported using condoms the first time.

Nonetheless, peer pressure and substance use was also part of the mix. Over sixty percent said their friends' sexual activity had influenced them, and nearly one in five were using drugs or drinking at the time. Nearly six in 10 "wanted to get it over with." And, substantial numbers had mixed feelings about their decision.

About one in four would change their first partner (25%) if they could, and a similar number (28%) regrets the decision to have sex altogether.

Chapter 14

Abstinence: A Personal Choice

What is abstinence?

Abstinence simply means not having sex; it means refraining from sexual intercourse. For most people, abstinence is the absence of sexual contact altogether.

How does abstinence work?

Abstinence prevents pregnancy because sexual intercourse does not take place. It involves refraining from any activity that leads to an exchange of body fluids.

Periodic abstinence is often used by couples who are practicing the fertility awareness method of birth control as a means of preventing pregnancy during the fertile period of a woman's cycle.

How effective is abstinence?

Abstinence prevents pregnancy 100% of the time. It is the most effective form of birth control.

About This Chapter: Information in this chapter is from "Abstinence." Reprinted with permission from the American Pregnancy Association, http://www.americanpregnancy.org, © 2003. All rights reserved.

What are the side effects or health risks of abstinence?

There are no side effects or health risks related to abstinence.

What about abstinence and sexually transmitted diseases (STDs)?

Abstinence prevents the transmission of sexually transmitted diseases 100% of the time.

What about teenagers and abstinence?

Relationships that involve sexual intercourse are filled with physical, emotional, and psychological risks. Abstinence provides teenagers the opportunity to avoid those risks.

Individuals who abstain from sexual intercourse during their teenage years tend to have fewer sexual partners in their future. Remaining abstinent as a teenager means that you will be less likely to have the following occur:

- Contract a sexually transmitted disease

- Become infertile

- Develop cancer of the cervix

- Experience an unplanned pregnancy

How can my partner get to know me?

Sexual intercourse is not the only way two people can get to know each other. Too often, people open this door for drawing closer to one another only to regret the decision later because they did not really know each other at all. Intimacy can be developed through a variety of means such as the following:

> ✔ **Quick Tip**
> ### How Can I Be Successful At Abstinence?
>
> Abstinence is most successful when you are diligent and use planning within your relationships. To make it easier, try some of the following ideas:
>
> - Do things with friends or in groups.
>
> - Go on double dates.
>
> - Minimize physical affection that could lead to passion and desire, making it harder to abstain from sexual intercourse.
>
> - Avoid situations where you are alone.
>
> For additional information, go to www.worththewait.org.

- Talking and listening

- Sharing joys, hurts, dreams, goals, wishes, and other aspects of life

- Honesty and respect for one another

- Having fun and playing together

For additional information, go to www.worththewait.org.

Why should someone choose abstinence?

Abstinence is chosen by women and men for a number of reasons. Some of the reasons people choose abstinence are noted below:

- Honor of personal, moral, or religious beliefs

- Waiting until they are married and in a monogamous and committed relationship

- Pursuing school, career, and other activities

- To avoid pregnancy and sexually transmitted diseases

For additional information, go to www.worththewait.org.

How can I express my affection?

Intimacy and affection can be expressed in a number of ways other than sexual intercourse. Kissing, hugging, massaging, and holding hands are some of the ways that couples express their affection in a physical manner. Intimacy and affection can also be expressed in other ways such as the following:

- Conversations

- Cards, letters, and love notes

- Support in your partner's activities

- Creative and fun dating (other than movies)

The caution with any physical affection is that it can lead to passion and a desire for something more.

What are the pros and cons of abstinence?

The pros of abstinence include the following:

- Has no side effects or health risks

- Prevents pregnancy and the transmission of sexually transmitted diseases

- Free

- Endorsed by many churches and religious organizations

- Reduces emotional and psychological challenges related to relationships that involve sexual activity

The cons of abstinence include the following:

- Requires willpower and discipline

Chapter 15

Masturbation

When you were really little, you may have learned that touching your body makes you feel good. A lot of you have probably stopped since then. Masturbation involves touching your penis or your clitoris, vulva or vagina in a way that gives you sexual pleasure. Exciting sexual thoughts fill your head, and, if you go long enough, you'll probably have an orgasm (rhythmic muscle contractions that produce a feeling of pleasure). Masturbation is a great way of giving yourself sexual pleasure, getting to know your body and what you like sexually, or just to burn off some sexual tension. It's also completely harmless and can give you a lot of sexual pleasure without the risk of pregnancy or getting a sexually transmitted infection.

These days, most people don't see masturbation as "wrong," provided it's done privately. But some religions may call masturbation immoral or a sin, and some parents may frown upon it. Masturbating is a great outlet for your body's sexual responses, but you're free to practice it or not. It's your choice, and it's completely up to you. If you are comfortable with it and you want to masturbate, do it. Just find a private place and a time when you're not going to be disturbed and give it a try. If you don't want to masturbate, or you think

About This Chapter: "Life After Puberty: Masturbation," is reprinted from www.sexualityandu.ca, with the permission of the Society of Obstetricians and Gynaecologists of Canada (SOGC). Users are forbidden to copy this material and/or redisseminate the data, in an original or modified form, for commercial purposes, without the expressed permission of SOGC. © 2007 www.sexualityandu.ca.

♣ **It's A Fact!!**

Is Masturbation Normal?

Masturbation (also called self pleasuring, "jerking off," or "playing with yourself") is a personal choice. Some people are comfortable touching themselves and some are not. Both are okay.

Masturbation is a normal activity that people may do alone or with a partner. It involves rubbing or touching your or your partner's body in a way that arouses sexual feelings and might produce an orgasm. Males and females of any age can masturbate.

Masturbation is not harmful. Most people see it as a normal part of sexuality. It can give pleasure, can be relaxing, help you sleep, and is an outlet for sexual tension. Masturbating may help to teach you about your own body and learn about where you like to be touched. You may choose to share this information with your partner. If a woman doesn't have orgasms easily, masturbation can help her learn how. Women more commonly experience orgasms through masturbation than through intercourse alone.

Some people do not masturbate because they don't get pleasure from it, or because they are uncomfortable touching their bodies. In some religions, masturbation is not acceptable. All of these choices are normal.

Masturbation is not acceptable if it is done in front of a person who has not wanted or permitted it.

There are a few things to keep in mind to make masturbation safer. Touching genitals with clean hands helps avoid spreading germs. Avoid putting a sharp or unclean object into a vagina or anus because it can cause tearing or infection. Any sex toys that are used during masturbation should not be shared with a partner without being cleaned first.

Source: Excerpted from "FAQs," from www.sexualityandu.ca, with the permission of the Society of Obstetricians and Gynaecologists of Canada (SOGC). Users are forbidden to copy this material and/or redisseminate the data, in an original or modified form, for commercial purposes, without the expressed permission of SOGC. © 2007 www.sexualityandu.ca.

it's wrong, that's perfectly fine too. The truth is, each person is different and people have to decide for themselves how they feel about it. But one thing you should know is that masturbation is very common and isn't going to harm you.

Guys usually masturbate by stroking and rubbing their penis, while girls usually rub or press around their clitoris with their hands or a comfortable object. Fantasizing about sex or something you find sexy may also help to enhance the experience. It's perfectly okay, and it's a great way to add to the pleasure of masturbation.

How you masturbate is a matter of whatever feels right for you—you can't masturbate "wrong." You'll probably find that you get better at it each time you do it. There's also no such thing as too much, but you might get sore if you rub a lot. And no, you won't go blind, you won't grow hair on your palms, your hands aren't going to fall off, and there is no such thing as a man running out of sperm. Masturbation also will not hurt your sex life later on. In fact, the things you learn about your own body now may actually help you be more comfortable when you decide you are ready for sex.

It may seem like guys talk about masturbating a lot more, but masturbating isn't just for guys, and it's not weird to be a girl who enjoys it. Millions upon millions of women masturbate. In addition to being really pleasurable, some women may not reach orgasm as easily as men, and masturbation is a good way for a woman to "practice" getting there. Knowing her body and knowing what feels good may help make sex better for her and her partner in the future. But again, masturbation is your choice to make. Do it if you want to, and don't if you don't. Some women may also masturbate to the point of orgasm as a way of soothing cramps during menstruation. Others, though, find that masturbating can make cramping worse.

Think of it this way. Whether or not you're having sex, masturbating helps you get to know your own body. It helps you figure out what turns you on, what feels good, and where you're sensitive. Once you know your own body well, you can tell or show your partner what you like best.

Chapter 16

Oral Sex: Is It Really Sex?

Can it cause pregnancy? Should you use condoms for it? Does having it make you lose your virginity?

Many teens are thinking about oral sex, and a new study by the National Center for Health Statistics (NCHS) found that more than half of U.S. teens ages 15 to 19 have done it—a much higher number than earlier studies had shown. What are the reasons behind this rising trend?

"Technical Virgins"

First, there's the idea of preserving virginity. Most teens agree that people lose their virginity the first time they have penile-vaginal intercourse. (Many also agree that people can lose their virginity through oral and anal sex if they have same-sex partners, but the NCHS study only asked teens about opposite-sex experiences.) To some teens, being a "technical virgin" is very important—they believe they can do everything but have vaginal sex and still remain a virgin.

The increasing importance of "technical virginity" is likely influenced by abstinence-only education, which focuses on teaching teens to avoid vaginal

About This Chapter: Information in this chapter is from "Examining Oral Sex," reprinted with permission from Planned Parenthood® Federation of America, Inc. © 2007 PPFA. All rights reserved. For additional information, visit www.plannedparenthood.org.

sex. "In abstinence education, you learn that you should stay a virgin," says Matt, 15. "So if you have oral sex, you don't have to lose your virginity, and you don't feel like you are doing something as bad."

Matt isn't the only teen who thinks oral sex "doesn't count." A Columbia University study found that teens who took virginity pledges were more likely to have anal and oral sex than teens who didn't pledge. Pledgers were substituting these other kinds of sex play for vaginal sex in order to stay "technical virgins."

The New Safer Sex?

Sarah, 19, thinks teens are having oral sex instead of vaginal sex because they believe it's safer. So is it? "There are fewer health risks for oral sex than there are for anal and vaginal sex, and pregnancy rates are down," says Nora Gelperin, director of training for the Network for Family Life Education in New Jersey, which publishes the website Sex, Etc. "Infection rates are up, which is not good, but we need to acknowledge that oral sex is less risky than other things."

♣ **It's A Fact!!**
Oral sex can't cause pregnancy, and it's very low risk for human immunodeficiency virus (HIV). However, oral sex can put both partners at risk for other sexually transmitted infections, including gonorrhea, herpes, human papillomavirus (HPV), and syphilis, among others. Using condoms to cover the penis or Glyde dams to cover the vulva or anus can reduce the risk of infection.

Do teens use protection for oral sex? "Never happened, never will," says Lisa, 15. Sarah agreed, saying the people she knows rarely use condoms for oral sex. And the NCHS study found the same—only nine percent of the teens surveyed reported using condoms for oral sex.

Since abstinence-only education doesn't teach about safer sex, many teens may not be aware of how to reduce their risk of infection during oral sex. "We need to look at how to help kids be informed and safe when they're engaged in this behavior," says Gelperin.

'Tis Better To Give Than Receive?

In the past, many people thought of oral sex as a one-way street—something girls would give and guys would get. "A lot of adults are concerned about the seeming inequity of girls performing oral sex on guys—that she's just being exploited by him," says Gelperin.

But according to the NCHS study, guys are giving and receiving oral sex at about the same rate as girls—even if they don't always tell their friends about it. "I think most guys like to give it if they get it," says Jabari, 17, "but they don't always like to talk about the fact that they like to give it."

Gelperin says she wasn't very surprised by the findings, since the study looked at older teens. "As teens mature, the relationships are a little more long-lasting, and the issue of reciprocity and equality in relationships becomes more important," she says.

The Bottom Line

As with any kind of sex play, communication is key when it comes to oral sex. Talking about safer sex, likes and dislikes, and what we're ready or not ready to do goes a long way towards making sex play enjoyable and comfortable for both people.

Chapter 17

Sexual Orientation And Homosexuality

What is sexual orientation?

Sexual orientation is an enduring emotional, romantic, sexual, or affectional attraction toward others. It is easily distinguished from other components of sexuality including biological sex, gender identity (the psychological sense of being male or female), and the social gender role (adherence to cultural norms for feminine and masculine behavior).

Sexual orientation exists along a continuum that ranges from exclusive heterosexuality to exclusive homosexuality and includes various forms of bi-sexuality. Bisexual persons can experience sexual, emotional, and affectional attraction to both their own sex and the opposite sex. Persons with a homo-sexual orientation are sometimes referred to as gay (both men and women) or as lesbian (women only).

Sexual orientation is different from sexual behavior because it refers to feelings and self-concept. Individuals may or may not express their sexual orientation in their behaviors.

What causes a person to have a particular sexual orientation?

There are numerous theories about the origins of a person's sexual orientation. Most scientists today agree that sexual orientation is most likely the result of a complex interaction of environmental, cognitive, and biological factors. In most people, sexual orientation is shaped at an early age. There is also considerable recent evidence to suggest that biology, including genetic or inborn hormonal factors, play a significant role in a person's sexuality.

It's important to recognize that there are probably many reasons for a person's sexual orientation, and the reasons may be different for different people.

Is sexual orientation a choice?

No. Human beings cannot choose to be either gay or straight. For most people, sexual orientation emerges in early adolescence without any prior sexual experience. Although we can choose whether to act on our feelings, psychologists do not consider sexual orientation to be a conscious choice that can be voluntarily changed.

Can therapy change sexual orientation?

No. Even though most homosexuals live successful, happy lives, some homosexual or bisexual people may seek to change their sexual orientation through therapy, often coerced by family members or religious groups to try and do so. The reality is that homosexuality is not an illness. It does not require treatment and is not changeable. However, not all gay, lesbian, and bisexual people who seek assistance from a mental health professional want to change their sexual orientation. Gay, lesbian, and bisexual people may seek psychological help with the coming out process or for strategies to deal with prejudice, but most go into therapy for the same reasons and life issues that bring straight people to mental health professionals.

What about so-called "conversion therapies"?

Some therapists who undertake so-called conversion therapy report that they have been able to change their clients' sexual orientation from homosexual to heterosexual. Close scrutiny of these reports, however, show several factors that cast doubt on their claims. For example, many of these claims come from organizations with an ideological perspective that condemns homosexuality. Furthermore, their claims are poorly documented; for example, treatment outcome is not followed and reported over time, as would be the standard to test the validity of any mental health intervention.

The American Psychological Association is concerned about such therapies and their potential harm to patients. In 1997, the Association's Council of Representatives passed a resolution reaffirming psychology's opposition to homophobia in treatment and spelling out a client's right to unbiased treatment and self-determination. Any person who enters into therapy to deal with issues of sexual orientation has a right to expect that such therapy will take place in a professionally neutral environment, without any social bias.

Is homosexuality a mental illness or emotional problem?

No. Psychologists, psychiatrists, and other mental health professionals agree that homosexuality is not an illness, a mental disorder, or an emotional problem. More than 35 years of objective, well-designed scientific research has shown that homosexuality, in and of itself, is not associated with mental disorders or emotional or social problems. Homosexuality was once thought to be a mental illness because mental health professionals and society had biased information.

In the past, the studies of gay, lesbian, and bisexual people involved only those in therapy, thus biasing the resulting conclusions. When researchers examined data about such people who were not in therapy, the idea that homosexuality was a mental illness was quickly found to be untrue.

In 1973 the American Psychiatric Association confirmed the importance of the new, better-designed research and removed homosexuality from the official manual that lists mental and emotional disorders. Two years later, the American Psychological Association passed a resolution supporting this removal.

For more than 25 years, both associations have urged all mental health professionals to help dispel the stigma of mental illness that some people still associate with homosexual orientation.

Can lesbians, gay men, and bisexuals be good parents?

Yes. Studies comparing groups of children raised by homosexual and by heterosexual parents find no developmental differences between the two groups of children in four critical areas: their intelligence, psychological adjustment, social adjustment, and popularity with friends. It is also important to realize that a parent's sexual orientation does not indicate their children's.

Another myth about homosexuality is the mistaken belief that gay men have more of a tendency than heterosexual men to sexually molest children. There is no evidence to suggest that homosexuals molest children.

Why do some gay men, lesbians, and bisexuals tell people about their sexual orientation?

Because sharing that aspect of themselves with others is important to their mental health. In fact, the process of identity development for lesbians, gay men, and bisexuals called "coming out" has been found to be strongly related to psychological adjustment; the more positive the gay, lesbian, or bisexual identity, the better one's mental health and the higher one's self-esteem.

Why is the "coming out" process difficult for some gay, lesbian, and bisexual people?

For some gay and bisexual people the "coming out" process is difficult; for others it is not. Often lesbian, gay, and bisexual people feel afraid, different, and alone when they first realize that their sexual orientation is different from the community norm. This is particularly true for people becoming aware of their gay, lesbian, or bisexual orientation in childhood or adolescence, which is not uncommon. And depending on their families and their communities, they may have to struggle against prejudice and misinformation about homosexuality.

Children and adolescents may be particularly vulnerable to the harmful effects of bias and stereotypes. They may also fear being rejected by family, friends, co-workers, and religious institutions. Some gay people have to worry about losing their jobs or being harassed at school if their sexual orientation became well known.

Unfortunately, gay, lesbian, and bisexual people are at a higher risk for physical assault and violence than are heterosexuals. Studies done in California in the mid-1990s showed that nearly one-fifth of all lesbians who took part in the study, and more than one-fourth of all gay men who participated, had been the victim of a hate crime based on their sexual orientation. In another California study of approximately 500 young adults, half of all the young men participating in the study admitted to some form of anti-gay aggression, ranging from name-calling to physical violence.

What can be done to overcome the prejudice and discrimination that gay men, lesbians, and bisexuals experience?

Research has found that the people who have the most positive attitudes toward gay men, lesbians, and bisexuals are those who say they know one or more gay, lesbian, or bisexual person well, often as a friend or co-worker. For this reason, psychologists believe that negative attitudes toward gay people as a group are prejudices that are not grounded in actual experience but are based on stereotypes and misinformation. Furthermore, protection against violence and discrimination are very important, just as they are for any other minority groups. Some states include violence against an individual on the basis of his or her sexual orientation as a "hate crime," and ten U.S. states have laws against discrimination on the basis of sexual orientation.

Why is it important for society to be better educated about homosexuality?

Educating all people about sexual orientation and homosexuality is likely to diminish anti-gay prejudice. Accurate information about homosexuality is especially important to young people who are first discovering and seeking to understand their sexuality, whether homosexual, bisexual, or heterosexual. Fears that access to such information will make more people gay have no validity; information about homosexuality does not make someone gay or straight.

Are all gay and bisexual men human immunodeficiency virus (HIV) infected?

No. This is a common myth. In reality, the risk of exposure to HIV is related to a person's behavior, not their sexual orientation. What's important to remember about human immunodeficiency virus/acquired immune deficiency syndrome (HIV/AIDS) is that contracting the disease can be prevented by using safe sex practices and by not using drugs.

Chapter 18

Transgender Individuals And Gender Identity

What does transgendered mean?

A transgendered (TG) person is someone whose gender identity (man or woman) does not match his or her biological sex (male or female). For most people, there is no incongruity between their biological sex and their internal gender identification. For TG people, their gender identity is in conflict with their biological sex.

Are there different types of transgendered individuals?

Yes. The term transgendered (TG) is an umbrella term used for many kinds of people with differing gender expression:

- **Transgendered:** The TG term is also used for someone who feels more comfortable as the other gender. TG individuals live part- or full-time as the other gender.

- **Transsexual:** Seeks to permanently change body to match her or his personal gender definition through gender reassignment surgery (GRS). "Non-op" refers to a person who has all the hormonal/surgical treatment except the GRS because he/she has no desire to proceed with the surgery, or cannot financially afford it.

About This Chapter: Information in this chapter is from "Understanding Transgender," by Jennifer Sager, M. Ed., © 2003 University of Florida Counseling Center. Reprinted with permission.

- **Transvestite:** Wears clothing of a gender opposite their birth sex for emotional or sexual purposes.

- **Two Spirited:** Having both female and male spirits (Native American culture). Often viewed with respect because they were able to hold both gender spirits in their bodies.

- **Intersexed or Hermaphrodite:** Rare medical condition where babies are born with both male and female sexual organs. Sex is assigned at birth.

Can people stop being transgendered?

No. People cannot change their gender identity. Gender identity is believed to be related to neuroanatomy, hormones, and/or genetics. Although some people will "give it up," they typically return to cross-dressing and recognize that they cannot fight their true nature.

Is gender identity not the same as sexual orientation?

- **Gender Identity:** Refers to how a person identifies as a man or a woman.

- **Sexual Orientation:** Refers to a romantic and sexual connection to a particular gender or genders (lesbian, gay, bisexual, or heterosexual).

A person's sexual orientation does not change after hormonal therapy or GRS. For example, when a genetic male, who is attracted to women, undergoes the GRS (thereby becoming a woman), she would call herself a lesbian. She now identifies as a woman (gender identity) who is attracted to other women (sexual orientation).

What if you think you are transgendered?

You may feel that you feel confused or don't know how to talk to your friends about this topic. It is important to explore your gender identity and seek help, whether that is through friends, family, counseling, support groups, or on-line chat rooms. Books, magazines, and web pages can help normalize your experience. Support from others will be important as you accept yourself.

What if you have a friend who is transgendered?

People want to be referred to in a language that represents their internal sense of self. Use the pronouns that are congruent with the gender they are presenting with. If someone close to you is TG, then ask her or him what pronoun you should use. In addition, ask if they are going to continue to use their birth name or if they have chosen a new name.

Where can you get support for being transgendered?

- Counseling can be beneficial as you learn to accept this part of yourself and tell friends and/or family.

- Support groups with other TG individuals will offer a community as you explore your gender identity.

- Gender specialists can assist you in the fine details of how to act in your new gender (for example, voice training).

- Consultation with someone who is familiar with transgendered issues can help guide you through medical and legal procedures.

✔ Quick Tip

National Support Groups

- International Foundation for Gender Education (IFGE)
- Society for the Second Self (Tri-Ess)
- Renaissance Transgender Association
- FTM International

Partner Support Groups

- Spouses and Partners International Conference for Education
- Crossdresser's Significant Others (CDSO)
- Rainbow Trail—Support for Family and Friends

Chapter 19

Sexuality In The Mass Media: How To View The Media Critically

The mass media has become an extremely pervasive and omnipresent institution, especially in American society. The Committee on Public Education reported last year that young people spend more time in front of the television than they do in school or with their parents, and by the time the average 18 year-old graduates from high school, he or she will have spent 15,000 hours watching television.

The changes in media representations of sex and sexuality over the last fifty years are astonishing. The media industries are no longer forced to portray husbands and wives occupying separate beds, and scenes of sexual activity are rarely avoided or quietly inferred. Sex in the mass media, especially on television, is becoming increasingly frequent and explicit, as many advertisers have come to the realization that "sex sells." Viewers can observe depictions of intimacy and affection, marriage and family life, and gender roles, as well as suggestive and erotic behavior, right in their living rooms.

On the one hand, the pervasive, accessible, and popular nature of television makes it an excellent instructor, offering an opportune way to learn about sex and sexuality without embarrassment. However, the images on television can be harmfully limited, stereotypical, and one-dimensional, depicting sex as an activity that is only acceptable for the young, single, and beautiful. Also, sex encounters may be continuously and erroneously presented as spontaneous, romantic, and risk-free.

How much sexual content is shown on television?

- About 66% of prime time shows contain some sexual content.

- In one study, a solid majority (62%) of scenes in television shows were coded as including some sexual behavior, and 28% of these scenes placed the primary emphasis on sex.

- Each new season television programs contain more sexual content than the previous year.

- Two thirds of the 1999–2000 television season contained some sexual content (up from one half the previous season).

- The sexual content of sitcom scenes shot up from 56% in 1999 to 84% in 2000.

- Eighty percent of the content presented on soap operas is sexual in nature, and there is an average of 6.6 sex acts in each soap hour.

- The television programs that are most popular with adolescents have been found to be the most sexual in nature.

How much sexual information do viewers utilize?

- Nearly 50% of adolescents report getting information about birth control from the mass media.

- Four out of ten teens (40%) report that they have gained ideas for how to talk to a boyfriend or girlfriend about sex directly from media portrayals.

- The mass media was the source of information about sexuality and relationships that was most frequently mentioned in a survey of youth ages ten to fifteen.

✤ It's A Fact!!

It is no longer possible, considering the enormous degree of media saturation in our culture, for the media to have zero effect on any aspect of human life, including human sexuality.

Who is having sex on television?

- Almost 23% of the sexual portrayals that were shown in the 2000 season involve characters from the ages of 18–24, and 9% (almost one in ten) involve characters under the age of 18.

- The bulk of the sexual action and language occurs between unmarried characters. One study found that unmarried heterosexual characters engage in sexual intercourse four to eight times as much as married characters.

- In one study of soap operas, there was only one representation of a married couple engaging in sex for every 24 portrayals of unmarried characters performing sexual acts.

How safe is sex on television?

- The use of contraceptives and the contraction of sexually transmitted diseases (STDs) on television are relatively rare. In one study, STDs were only mentioned an average of once every ten program hours. In this study, even when a reference was made to the risk of sexual behavior, it was very rarely the primary emphasis of the scene.

- Nearly 14,000 sexual references bombard the average American adolescent each year, yet only "165 of these will deal with birth control, self-control, abstinence, or the risk of pregnancy or STDs."

What are some possible effects of increased exposure to mass media sexuality?

- Several studies have linked increased exposure to the mass media with dissatisfaction with virginity among teenagers.

- The students who think television accurately portrays sex were more likely to be dissatisfied with their first experience with intercourse.

- Teens that had been exposed to a highly sexual television drama rated descriptions of casual sex encounters less negatively than teens that had received no sexual content exposure.

♣ **It's A Fact!!**
Many people are being exposed to massive and explicit sexual messages every day of their lives, probably beginning before they have the knowledge or sophistication to accurately deal with such complicated content.

- A study of black women aged 14 to 18 revealed that adolescents who see X-rated movies have less favorable attitudes toward condom use than other teens.

None of these statistics or research findings indicate that watching sexual content on television makes viewers take irresponsible steps in their own lives. The research does, however, point to the notion that television viewing may help shape viewers' attitudes and expectations about sexual relationships, which, in turn, are some of the strongest predictors of their behavior. This hypothesis links sexual attitudes developed from the media with troubling sexual statistics, such as the fact that the United States has a higher rate of teen pregnancy than any other industrialized country in the world.

What is the good news?

However, the media may help break down the cultural taboos associated with sensitive sexual topics and bridge gaps in our sexual knowledge. Daytime talk shows and television movies reveal a wide range of human sexual expression and broach topics such as rape, incest, and abortion. An organization called The Media Project works with the television industry to incorporate realistic information about human sexuality and responsibility into their programming. The Media Project even sponsors the annual SHINE Awards (Sexual Health In Entertainment) to recognize mass media outlets that have constructively portrayed sexual issues to the public.

Because the media can be a double-edged sword, delivering both entertainment and harmful messages, it is important to view sexual media critically.

The following are some tips and ideas to help you evaluate the media more carefully and critically.

Questions that will assist in critical viewing are the following:

- Who has created the sexual images?

- Who is engaging in the sexual behavior?

- Whose viewpoint is not heard?

- From whose perspective does the camera frame the events?

- How would your parents, girlfriend, or boyfriend talk about the story you just saw?

- What is our role as spectators in identifying with, or questioning what we see and hear?

- Who owns the medium? How much do the owners profit from showing sexual content?

Tips on viewing sexualized advertisements, movies, and television shows are as follows:

- Watch together. You not only learn about the content, but how others are reacting to it.

- Dialogue and listen to what others say about sexual content on television.

- Learn to read sexualized advertisements. What's the message? Who is the ad targeting? What are they using to make the ad appeal to their target audience? How much are they spending to convince their target audience to buy that product?

- Test an ad's claims (does a certain perfume actually make the wearer more sexy or attractive?). Be creative.

- Develop rules for watching and guidelines for choosing sexual movies and videos.

- Dialogue and listen to what others are saying about sexual images in movies and videos.

- Learn about and utilize the Motion Picture Rating System.

- Learn about and utilize the TV Rating System.

Chapter 20

Rape And Date Rape: What You Should Know

What is rape and date rape?

Rape is sex you do not agree to, including forcing a body part or object into your vagina, rectum (bottom), or mouth. Date rape is when you are raped by someone you know. Both are crimes. Rape is not about sex; it is an act of power by the rapist, and it is always wrong.

Date rape drugs, which often have no smell or taste, can be given to you without you knowing at parties or in a club, especially where alcohol is served. Alcohol can make you less aware of danger and make you less able to think clearly and resist sexual assault. If you are given date rape drugs, you may not be able to say "no" to unwanted sex, and you may not be able to clearly remember what happened.

What should I know about date rape drugs?

Date rape drugs are most commonly used to sexually assault a person. The drugs often have no color, smell, or taste and are easily added to drinks without the victim's knowledge. These drugs usually cause a person to become helpless; they can hardly move and are not able to protect themselves

About This Chapter: Information in this chapter is from "What is rape and date rape?" GirlsHealth.gov, sponsored by the National Women's Health Information Center, U.S. Department of Health and Human Services, August 2006.

> ☞ **Remember!!**
> Even if you were drinking, it is not your fault.

from being hurt. People who have been given date rape drugs say they felt paralyzed or could not see well, and had blackouts, problems talking, confusion, and dizziness. Date rape drugs can even cause death.

It is hard to know whether a party, club, or concert you plan to go to will be dangerous. Drugs may not be at every party you go to, but you should still have a plan for keeping yourself and your friends safe no matter what. The following are some things to remember:

- Say "no" to alcohol. Have water or soda instead.

- Open your own drinks.

- Do not let other people hand you drinks.

- Keep your drink with you at all times, even when you go to the bathroom.

- Do not share drinks.

- Do not drink from punch bowls or other large, common, open containers. They may already have drugs in them.

- Do not drink anything that tastes, looks, or smells strange. Sometimes, GHB [gamma-hydroxybutyrate] tastes salty.

- Always go to a party, club, or concert with someone you trust, such as a friend or an older brother or sister.

I think I was raped. What should I do?

- Do not blame yourself. The rape was not your fault.

- Get help right away. Call the National Sexual Assault Hotline at 1-800-656-HOPE (4673) for help or go to the police or local hospital. You may want to take a friend or family member along for support.

- If possible, do not urinate before getting help. Your urine can help show signs of the rape.

- Do not douche, bathe, or change clothes before getting help. Doing these things can remove possible evidence of the rape, such as semen (fluid from a man) or hair belonging to the person who assaulted you.

- Get medical care right away. Tell the doctor or nurse if you think you were drugged. He or she will give you a urine test right away because date rape drugs leave your body quickly. You will also get a medical exam to make sure you do not have other injuries. The doctor or nurse will test you for sexually transmitted diseases (STDs), including human immunodeficiency virus/acquired immunodeficiency syndrome (HIV/AIDS), and offer you emergency contraception to prevent pregnancy. If the doctor or nurse does not mention testing for STDs or emergency contraception, ask for them.

- The counselor will help you figure out how to tell your parents/guardians. They may be angry or upset, but only because they care about you and do not want you to get hurt. Getting help and dealing with your emotions is the first step in healing.

Whom can I call for help?

There are free hotlines that you can call 24 hours a day to get help if you have been sexually assaulted or if you need advice on how to leave an unhealthy relationship.

- National Sexual Assault Hotline: 1-800-656-HOPE (4673)

- National Domestic Violence Hotline: 1-800-799-SAFE (7233) or 1-800-787-3224 (TTY)

- Girls and Boys Town National Hotline: 1-800-448-3000 or 1-800-448-1833 (TTY)

You can also find local resources, including women's shelters or other services through your religious center, school, or doctor's office.

Chapter 21

Protecting Yourself From Online Sexual Predators

The internet has opened up a whole new world for people of all ages. You can shop, plan a vacation, send a picture to a relative, talk with friends, and even do research for school. This new way of finding information and communicating does come with risks.

Safe Chatting

What kind of online name should I choose?

You should never use your real name as your online name. By using your real name, anyone can know right away who you are and can probably find out more about you. This is especially true in chat rooms, where you can get comfortable chatting with someone and suddenly realize they know things about you.

You probably want your online name to describe who you are, but be careful about the name and words you choose. Remember, when you are talking online to people you do not know well, some people may unfairly judge you by your online name. For example, if you choose a name like

About This Chapter: Information in this chapter is from "Safety on the Internet," "Safe Chatting," and "Safe Blogging," GirlsHealth.gov, sponsored by the National Women's Health Information Center, U.S. Department of Health and Human Services, August 2006.

hotbabe13, people will get the wrong idea about you, and you most likely will get unwanted e-mails from people who are just responding to your online name and not to who you really are. If you cannot think of an online name to use without describing something about yourself, try using the name of a candy bar, color, or something else that is not personal. If the name is already taken, you can try adding a few numbers, for example, Green123.

Is IMing safe?

IMing is not as private as you might think, so it is important to know how to stay safe and have fun too. Here are some tips:

☞ Remember!!

Before you enter a chat, be sure you have permission from a parent or guardian to do so.

Source: Excerpted from "Safe Chatting," GirlsHealth.gov.

• Do not respond to IMs from people you do not know or IMs that look strange. It is possible to get unwanted IMs. Like e-mails, IMs can also contain viruses.

• Do not forget to sign off when you are finished and change your password regularly. This will keep others from using your IM account.

• If you get an IM that makes you feel uncomfortable, do not respond to it. Tell your parents/guardians about it.

• Never give out your screen name or password, even to your friends.

Are chat rooms safe?

Some chat rooms are thought to be safe because the topic that is being talked about is safe, and because there is a moderator leading the chat. Even if the topic is okay, some people might talk about other things that can make you uncomfortable. If you ever feel uncomfortable or in danger for any reason, leave the chat room right away and tell a parent/guardian or other trusted adult.

Can the chat moderator make sure nothing bad happens in the chat room?

A chat moderator supervises a chat. A moderator can kick someone out of a chat if they write something they shouldn't, but the moderator cannot stop you from going to a private chat area with someone who might harm or threaten you. If you are allowed to go to a chat, be careful to check out the topic first. Your parents/guardians can check out the chat room first to make sure the conversation is okay. Some people who go into chats may want to imagine that you are someone you are not or play out their fantasy by saying bad things to you. If anyone makes you feel uncomfortable, leave the chat immediately.

Safe Blogging

Is it safe to post a profile on MySpace, Friendster, or Facebook?

Many young people think the information they post on social networking sites such as MySpace, Friendster, or Facebook will only be seen by their friends; often, this is not the case. Anything you post on a social networking site, even if it is in a "private" area, can be seen by almost anyone, including your parents/guardians, your teachers, employers, and strangers, some of whom could be dangerous. For this reason, you should not post information about yourself. Even information that seems harmless, such as where you went to dinner last night, could be used by a stranger to find you.

You should also be careful when looking through networking sites. Scam artists have been known to use personal information from your profile to pose as a friend, in hopes that you will give them personal information, such as your credit card or cell phone numbers. Never give out any personal information online. Here are some tips to follow:

- **Before joining a social networking site, think about who might be able to see your profile.** Some sites will let only certain users see your posted content; others let everyone see postings.

- **Think about keeping some control over the information you post.** If you can, limit access to your page to a select group of people such as your friends from school, your club, your team, your community groups, or your family. Keep in mind, though, this does not always mean that other people cannot see your page.

- **Keep your information to yourself.** Do not post your full name, social security number, address, phone number, or bank and credit card account numbers, and do not post other people's information either. Be careful about posting information that could be used to identify you or locate you offline. This could include the name of your school, sports team, clubs, and where you work or hang out.

- **Make sure your screen name does not say too much about you.** Do not use your name, your age, or your hometown. It does not take a genius to combine clues to figure out who you are and where you can be found.

- **Post only information that you are comfortable with others seeing, and knowing, about you.** Many people can see your page, including your parents/guardians, your teachers, the police, the college you might want to apply to next year, or the job you might want to apply for in five years.

- **Remember that once you post information online, you cannot take it back.** Even if you delete the information from a site, older versions exist on other people's computers.

- **Do not post your photo.** It can be changed and spread around in ways you may not be happy about.

- **Do not flirt with strangers online.** Because some people lie about whom they really are, you never really know whom you are dealing with.

- **Do not meet someone you met online in person.** If someone you met online wants to meet you in person, tell your parents/guardians or a trusted adult right away.

🖝 Remember!!

Do not post your photo on the internet or send it to someone you do not know.

Do not post or send personal information including the following:

- full name
- address
- phone number
- login name, IM screen name, passwords
- school name
- school location
- sports teams
- clubs
- city you live in
- social security number
- financial information (credit card numbers and bank account numbers)
- where you work or hang out
- names of family members

Source: Excerpted from "Safe Blogging," GirlsHealth.gov.

- **Trust your gut if you have suspicions.** If you feel threatened by someone or uncomfortable because of something online, tell your parents/guardians or an adult you trust and report it to the police and the website. You could end up protecting someone else.

Is it okay to share my password with my best friend?

No. You should not share your password with any of your friends, even your best friend. The only people who should know your internet or e-mail password are your parents/guardians and you. If you let someone else know what your password is, then they can read anything that you may want to keep private. Another person could use bad language or go to sites you should not be visiting under your name.

Is there anything that I shouldn't tell someone on the internet?

Yes. Just like you would not walk up to a stranger and give out your phone number or share your name, where you live, or where you go to school, you should not share this kind of information online either. It is very important that you do not e-mail or IM anyone that you do not know or share any information that can identify you.

Part Three

For Girls Only

Chapter 22

The Female Reproductive System: An Overview

The organs of the female reproductive system produce and sustain the female sex cells (egg cells or ova), transport these cells to a site where they may be fertilized by sperm, provide a favorable environment for the developing fetus, move the fetus to the outside at the end of the development period, and produce the female sex hormones.

♣ **It's A Fact!!**
The female reproductive system includes the ovaries, fallopian tubes, uterus, vagina, accessory glands, and external genital organs.

Source: "Reproductive System," SEER's Training Web Site, 2000.

Ovaries

The primary female reproductive organs, or gonads, are the two ovaries. Each ovary is a solid, ovoid structure about the size and shape of an almond, about 3.5 cm in length, 2 cm wide, and 1 cm thick. The ovaries are located in shallow depressions, called ovarian fossae, one on each side of the uterus, in the lateral walls of the pelvic cavity. They are held loosely in place by peritoneal ligaments.

About This Chapter: Information in this chapter is from "Reproductive System," from the National Cancer Institute's Surveillance, Epidemiology and End Results (SEER) Training Web Site, 2000. Note: Despite the older date of this document, the anatomical information it presents is still current.

Structure

The ovaries are covered on the outside by a layer of simple cuboidal epithelium called germinal (ovarian) epithelium. This is actually the visceral peritoneum that envelops the ovaries. Underneath this layer there

is a dense connective tissue capsule, the tunica albuginea. The substance of the ovaries is distinctly divided into an outer cortex and an inner medulla. The cortex appears more dense and granular due to the presence of numerous ovarian follicles in various stages of development. Each of the follicles contains an oocyte, a female germ cell. The medulla is loose connective tissue with abundant blood vessels, lymphatic vessels, and nerve fibers.

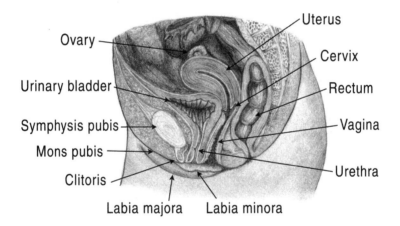

Figure 22.1. Organs of the Female Reproductive System

Oogenesis

Female sex cells, or gametes, develop in the ovaries by a form of meiosis called oogenesis. The sequence of events in oogenesis is similar to the sequence in spermatogenesis, but the timing and final result is different. Early in fetal development, primitive germ cells in the ovaries differentiate into oogonia. These divide rapidly to form thousands of cells, still called oogonia, which have a full complement of 46 (23 pairs) chromosomes. Oogonia then enter a growth phase, enlarge, and become primary oocytes. The diploid (46 chromosomes) primary oocytes replicate their DNA and begin the first meiotic division, but the process stops in prophase and the cells remain in this suspended state until puberty. Many of the primary oocytes degenerate before birth, but even with this decline, the two ovaries together contain approximately 700,000 oocytes at birth. This is the lifetime supply, and no more will develop. This is quite different than the male in which spermatogonia and primary spermatocytes continue to be produced throughout the reproductive lifetime. By puberty the number of primary oocytes has further declined to about 400,000.

Beginning at puberty, under the influence of follicle-stimulating hormone, several primary oocytes start to grow again each month. One of the primary oocytes seems to outgrow the others, and it resumes meiosis I. The other cells degenerate. The large cell undergoes an unequal division so that nearly all the cytoplasm, organelles, and half the chromosomes go to one cell, which becomes a secondary oocyte. The remaining half of the chromosomes goes to a smaller cell called the first polar body. The secondary oocyte begins the second meiotic division, but the process stops in metaphase. At this point ovulation occurs. If fertilization occurs, meiosis II continues. Again this is an unequal division with all of the cytoplasm going to the ovum, which has 23 single-stranded chromosomes. The smaller cell from this division is a second polar body. The first polar body also usually divides in meiosis I to produce two even smaller polar bodies. If fertilization does not occur, the second meiotic division is never completed and the secondary oocyte degenerates. Here again, there are obvious differences between the male and female. In spermatogenesis, four functional sperm develop from each primary spermatocyte. In oogenesis, only one functional fertilizable cell develops from a primary oocyte. The other three cells are polar bodies and they degenerate.

Ovarian Follicle Development

An ovarian follicle consists of a developing oocyte surrounded by one or more layers of cells called follicular cells. At the same time that the oocyte is progressing through meiosis, corresponding changes are taking place in the follicular cells. Primordial follicles, which consist of a primary oocyte surrounded by a single layer of flattened cells, develop in the fetus and are the stage that is present in the ovaries at birth and throughout childhood.

Beginning at puberty follicle-stimulating hormone stimulates changes in the primordial follicles. The follicular cells become cuboidal, the primary oocyte enlarges, and it is now a primary follicle. The follicles continue to grow under the influence of follicle-stimulating hormone, and the follicular cells proliferate to form several layers of granulose cells around the primary oocyte. Most of these primary follicles degenerate along with the primary oocytes within them, but usually one continues to develop each month. The granulosa cells start secreting estrogen and a cavity, or antrum, forms within the follicle. When the antrum starts to develop, the follicle becomes a secondary follicle. The granulose cells also secrete a glycoprotein substance that forms a clear membrane, the zona pellucida, around the oocyte. After about 10 days of growth, the follicle is a mature vesicular (graafian) follicle, which forms a "blister" on the surface of the ovary and contains a secondary oocyte ready for ovulation.

Ovulation

Ovulation, prompted by luteinizing hormone from the anterior pituitary, occurs when the mature follicle at the surface of the ovary ruptures and releases the secondary oocyte into the peritoneal cavity. The ovulated secondary oocyte, ready for fertilization, is still surrounded by the zona pellucida and a few layers of cells called the corona radiata. If it is not fertilized, the secondary oocyte degenerates in a couple of days. If a sperm passes through the corona radiata and zona pellucida and enters the cytoplasm of the secondary oocyte, the second meiotic division resumes to form a polar body and a mature ovum.

After ovulation and in response to luteinizing hormone, the portion of the follicle that remains in the ovary enlarges and is transformed into a corpus luteum. The corpus luteum is a glandular structure that secretes progesterone and some estrogens. Its fate depends on whether fertilization occurs. If fertilization does not take place, the corpus luteum remains functional for about 10 days, and then it begins to degenerate into a corpus albicans, which is primarily scar tissue, and its hormone output ceases. If fertilization occurs, the corpus luteum persists and continues its hormone functions until the placenta develops sufficiently to secrete the necessary hormones. Again, the corpus luteum ultimately degenerates into corpus albicans, but it remains functional for a longer period of time.

Genital Tract

Fallopian Tubes

There are two uterine tubes, also called fallopian tubes or oviducts. There is one tube associated with each ovary. The end of the tube near the ovary expands to form a funnel-shaped infundibulum, which is surrounded by finger-like extensions called fimbriae. Because there is no direct connection between the infundibulum and the ovary, the oocyte enters the peritoneal cavity before it enters the fallopian tube. At the time of ovulation, the fimbriae increase their activity and create currents in the peritoneal fluid that help propel the oocyte into the fallopian tube. Once inside the fallopian tube, the oocyte is moved along by the rhythmic beating of cilia on the epithelial lining and by peristaltic action of the smooth muscle in the wall of the tube. The journey through the fallopian tube takes about 7 days. Because the oocyte is fertile for only 24 to 48 hours, fertilization usually occurs in the fallopian tube.

Uterus

The uterus is a muscular organ that receives the fertilized oocyte and provides an appropriate environment for the developing fetus. Before the first pregnancy, the uterus is about the size and shape of a pear, with the narrow portion directed inferiorly. After childbirth, the uterus is usually larger, and then regresses after menopause.

The uterus is lined with the endometrium. The stratum functionale of the endometrium sloughs off during menstruation. The deeper stratum basale provides the foundation for rebuilding the stratum functionale.

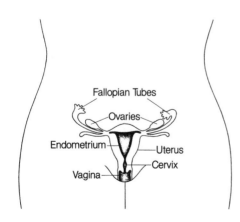

Figure 22.2. Uterus

Vagina

The vagina is a fibromuscular tube, about 10 cm long, that extends from the cervix of the uterus to the outside. It is located between the rectum and the urinary bladder. Because the vagina is tilted posteriorly as it ascends and the cervix is tilted anteriorly, the cervix projects into the vagina at nearly a right angle.

External Genitalia

The external genitalia are the accessory structures of the female reproductive system that are external to the vagina. They are also referred to as the vulva or pudendum. The external genitalia include the labia majora, mons pubis, labia minora, clitoris, and glands within the vestibule.

The clitoris is an erectile organ, similar to the male penis, that responds to sexual stimulation. Posterior to the clitoris, the urethra, vagina, paraurethral glands, and greater vestibular glands open into the vestibule.

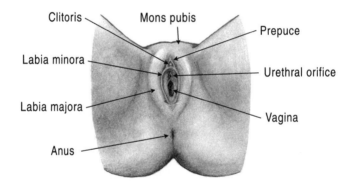

Figure 22.3. Female External Genitalia

Female Sexual Response And Hormone Control

The female sexual response includes arousal and orgasm, but there is no ejaculation. A woman may become pregnant without having an orgasm.

Follicle-stimulating hormone, luteinizing hormone, estrogen, and progesterone have major roles in regulating the functions of the female reproductive system.

At puberty, when the ovaries and uterus are mature enough to respond to hormonal stimulation, certain stimuli cause the hypothalamus to start secreting gonadotropin-releasing hormone. This hormone enters the blood and goes to the anterior pituitary gland where it stimulates the secretion of follicle-stimulating hormone and luteinizing hormone. These hormones, in turn, affect the ovaries and uterus and the monthly cycles begin. A woman's reproductive cycles last from menarche to menopause.

The monthly ovarian cycle begins with the follicle development during the follicular phase, continues with ovulation during the ovulatory phase, and concludes with the development and regression of the corpus luteum during the luteal phase.

The uterine cycle takes place simultaneously with the ovarian cycle. The uterine cycle begins with menstruation during the menstrual phase, continues with repair of the endometrium during the proliferative phase, and ends with the growth of glands and blood vessels during the secretory phase.

Menopause occurs when a woman's reproductive cycles stop. Decreased levels of ovarian hormones and increased levels of pituitary follicle-stimulating hormone and luteinizing hormone mark this period. The changing hormone levels are responsible for the symptoms associated with menopause.

Mammary Glands

Functionally, the mammary glands produce milk; structurally, they are modified sweat glands. Mammary glands, which are located in the breast overlying the pectoralis major muscles, are present in both sexes, but usually are functional only in the female.

Externally, each breast has a raised nipple, which is surrounded by a circular pigmented area called the areola. The nipples are sensitive to touch, due to the fact that they contain smooth muscle that contracts and causes them to become erect in response to stimulation.

✎ **What's It Mean?**

Chromosome: One of the linear, or sometimes circular DNA-containing bodies of viruses, prokaryotic organisms, and the cell nucleus of eukaryotic organisms, which contain most or all of the genes of the individual.

Estrogen: Any of various natural steroids that are secreted chiefly by the ovaries, placenta, adipose tissue, and testes, and that stimulate the development of female secondary sex characteristics and promote the growth and maintenance of the female reproductive system.

Fetus: A developing human from usually three months after conception to birth.

Source: SEER'S Training Web Site Glossary, available at http://training.seer.cancer.gov/stws_glossary.html; cited March 2007.

Internally, the adult female breast contains 15 to 20 lobes of glandular tissue that radiate around the nipple. The lobes are separated by connective tissue and adipose. The connective tissue helps support the breast. Some bands of connective tissue, called suspensory (Cooper's) ligaments extend through the breast from the skin to the underlying muscles. The amount and distribution of the adipose tissue determines the size and shape of the breast. Each lobe consists of lobules that contain the glandular units. A lactiferous duct collects the milk from the lobules within each lobe and carries it to the nipple. Just before the nipple, the lactiferous duct enlarges to form a lactiferous sinus (ampulla), which serves as a reservoir for milk. After the sinus, the duct again narrows and each duct opens independently on the surface of the nipple.

Hormones regulate mammary gland function. At puberty, increasing levels of estrogen stimulate the development of glandular tissue in the female breast. Estrogen also causes the breast to increase in size through the accumulation of adipose tissue. Progesterone stimulates the development of the duct system. During pregnancy these hormones enhance further development of the mammary glands. Prolactin from the anterior pituitary stimulates the production of milk within the glandular tissue, and oxytocin causes the ejection of milk from the glands.

Chapter 23

Menstruation And The Menstrual Cycle

Menstruation

What is menstruation?

Menstruation is a woman's monthly bleeding. It is also called menses, menstrual period, or period. When a woman has her period, she is menstruating. The menstrual blood is partly blood and partly tissue from the inside of the uterus (womb). It flows from the uterus through the small opening in the cervix and passes out of the body through the vagina. Most menstrual periods last from three to five days.

What is the menstrual cycle?

Menstruation is part of the menstrual cycle, which helps a woman's body prepare for the possibility of pregnancy each month. A cycle starts on the first day of a period. The average menstrual cycle is 28 days long. However, a cycle can range anywhere from 23 days to 35 days.

About This Chapter: This chapter begins with "Menstruation," from "Menstruation and the Menstrual Cycle," The National Women's Health Information Center, U.S. Department of Health and Human Services, Office on Women's Health, November 2002. Information under the heading "Amenorrhea," is from "Amenorrhea," National Institute of Child Health and Human Development, National Institutes of Health, May 2007. Text under the heading "Dysmenorrhea," is from "Dysmenorrhea (Painful Periods)," © 2005 Washington State University Health and Wellness Services. Reprinted with permission.

The parts of the body involved in the menstrual cycle include the brain, pituitary gland, uterus and cervix, ovaries, fallopian tubes, and vagina. Body chemicals, called hormones, rise and fall during the month and make the menstrual cycle happen. The ovaries make two important female hormones, estrogen and progesterone. Other hormones involved in the menstrual cycle include follicle-stimulating hormone (FSH) and luteinizing hormone (LH), made by the pituitary gland.

What happens during the menstrual cycle?

In the first half of the menstrual cycle, levels of estrogen rise and make the lining of the uterus grow and thicken. In response to follicle-stimulating hormone, an egg (ovum) in one of the ovaries starts to mature. At about day 14 of a typical 28-day cycle, in response to a surge of luteinizing hormone, the egg leaves the ovary. This is called ovulation.

In the second half of the menstrual cycle, the egg begins to travel through the fallopian tube to the uterus. Progesterone levels rise and help prepare the uterine lining for pregnancy. If the egg becomes fertilized by a sperm cell and attaches itself to the uterine wall, the woman becomes pregnant. If the egg is not fertilized, it either dissolves or is absorbed into the body. If pregnancy does not occur, estrogen and progesterone levels drop, and the thickened lining of the uterus is shed during the menstrual period.

What is a typical menstrual period like?

During the menstrual period, the thickened uterine lining and extra blood are shed through the vaginal canal. A woman's period may not be the same every month, and it may not be the same as other women's periods. Periods can be light, moderate, or heavy, and the length of the period also varies. While most menstrual periods last from three to five days, anywhere from two to seven days is considered normal. For the first few years after menstruation begins, periods may be very irregular. They may also become irregular in women approaching menopause. Sometimes birth control pills are prescribed to help with irregular periods or other problems with the menstrual cycle.

Sanitary pads or tampons, which are made of cotton or another absorbent material, are worn to absorb the blood flow. Sanitary pads are placed inside the panties; tampons are inserted into the vagina.

What kinds of problems do women have with their periods?

Women can have various kinds of problems with their periods, including pain, heavy bleeding, and skipped periods.

- **Amenorrhea:** The lack of a menstrual period. This term is used to describe the absence of a period in young women who have not started menstruating by age 16 or the absence of a period in women who used to have a regular period. Causes of amenorrhea include pregnancy, breastfeeding, and extreme weight loss caused by serious illness, eating disorders, excessive exercising, or stress. Hormonal problems (involving the pituitary, thyroid, ovary, or adrenal glands) or problems with the reproductive organs may be involved.

- **Dysmenorrhea:** Painful periods, including severe menstrual cramps. In younger women, there is often no known disease or condition associated with the pain. A hormone called prostaglandin is responsible for the symptoms. Some pain medicines available over the counter, such as ibuprofen, can help with these symptoms. Sometimes a disease or condition, such as uterine fibroids or endometriosis, causes the pain. Treatment depends on what is causing the problem and how severe it is.

♣ It's A Fact!!

Menarche is another name for the beginning of menstruation. In the United States, the average age a girl starts menstruating is 12. However, this does not mean that all girls start at the same age. A girl can begin menstruating anytime between the ages of 8 and 16. Menstruation will not occur until all parts of a girl's reproductive system have matured and are working together.

Source: "Menstruation and the Menstrual Cycle," The National Women's Health Information Center.

- **Abnormal Uterine Bleeding:** Vaginal bleeding that is different from normal menstrual periods. It includes very heavy bleeding or unusually long periods (also called menorrhagia), periods too close together, and bleeding between periods. In adolescents and women approaching menopause, hormone imbalance problems often cause menorrhagia along with irregular cycles. Sometimes this is called dysfunctional uterine bleeding (DUB). Other causes of abnormal bleeding include uterine fibroids and polyps. Treatment for abnormal bleeding depends on the cause.

When should I see a health care provider about my period?

You should consult your health care provider for the following:

- If you have not started menstruating by the age of 16.

- If your period has suddenly stopped.

- If you are bleeding for more days than usual.

- If you are bleeding excessively.

- If you suddenly feel sick after using tampons.

- If you bleed between periods (more than just a few drops).

- If you have severe pain during your period.

How often should I change my pad/tampon?

Sanitary napkins (pads) should be changed as often as necessary, before the pad is soaked with menstrual flow. Each woman decides for herself what is comfortable. Tampons should be changed

✔ **Quick Tip**
The Food and Drug Administration (FDA) recommends the following tips to help avoid tampon problems:

- Follow package directions for insertion.

- Choose the lowest absorbency for your flow.

- Change your tampon at least every 4 to 8 hours.

- Consider alternating pads with tampons.

- Know the warning signs of toxic shock syndrome [see Chapter 31 for more information].

- Do not use tampons between periods.

Source: "Menstruation and the Menstrual Cycle," The National Women's Health Information Center.

often (at least every 4–8 hours). Make sure that you use the lowest absorbency of tampon needed for your flow. For example, do not use super absorbency on the lightest day of your period. This can put you at risk for toxic shock syndrome (TSS). TSS is a rare but potentially deadly disease. Women under 30, especially teenagers, are at a higher risk for TSS. Using any kind of tampon—cotton or rayon of any absorbency—puts a woman at greater risk for TSS than using menstrual pads. The risk of TSS can be lessened or avoided by not using tampons or by alternating between tampons and pads during your period.

If you experience any of the following symptoms while you are menstruating and using tampons, you should contact your health care provider immediately: high fever that appears suddenly; muscle aches; diarrhea; dizziness and/or fainting; sunburn-like rash; sore throat; bloodshot eyes.

Amenorrhea

What is amenorrhea?

Amenorrhea is the absence of a menstrual period.

Primary amenorrhea is when a young woman has not yet had a period by age 16.

Secondary amenorrhea describes someone who used to have a regular period but then it stopped for at least three months (this can include pregnancy).

What are the signs of amenorrhea?

The main sign of amenorrhea is missing a menstrual period.

Regular periods are a sign of overall good health. Missing a period may mean that you are pregnant or that something is going wrong. It is important to tell your health care provider if you miss a period so he or she can begin to find out what is happening in your body.

Amenorrhea itself is not a disease but is usually a symptom of another condition. Depending on that condition, a woman might experience other symptoms, such as headache, vision changes, hair loss, or excess facial hair.

What are the causes of amenorrhea?

Amenorrhea is a symptom of a variety of conditions, ranging from not serious to serious.

Primary Amenorrhea

- Chromosomal or genetic abnormalities can cause the eggs and follicles involved in menstruation to deplete too early in life.

- Hypothalamic or pituitary diseases and physical problems, such as problems with reproductive organs, can prevent periods from starting.

- Moderate or excessive exercise, eating disorders (such as anorexia nervosa), extreme physical or psychological stress, or a combination of these can disrupt the normal menstrual cycle.

Secondary Amenorrhea

- This problem is much more common than primary amenorrhea.

- Common causes include many of those listed for primary amenorrhea, as well as pregnancy, certain contraceptives, breastfeeding, mental stress, and certain medications.

- Hormonal problems involving the hypothalamus, pituitary, thyroid, ovary, or adrenal glands can also cause amenorrhea.

- Women who have very low body weight sometimes stop getting their periods as well.

- Women with premature ovarian failure stop getting regular periods before natural menopause.

What is treatment for amenorrhea?

Treatment for amenorrhea depends on the underlying cause. Sometimes lifestyle changes can help if weight, stress, or physical activity is causing the amenorrhea. Other times medications and oral contraceptives can help the problem. For more information, talk to your health care provider.

Dysmenorrhea

Dysmenorrhea (pronounced dis-men-or-ree-a) is the medical term for menstrual periods that are painful or difficult. Symptoms include cramping pain in your abdomen, low back, and thighs, dizziness, headaches, nausea, and diarrhea. These symptoms of dysmenorrhea are usually the worst on the first day of your period and ease as your period continues. In most cases, they are gone after 12 to 16 hours. However, a woman's symptoms can last throughout her period.

Is dysmenorrhea "all in my head?"

No. Dysmenorrhea is a physical problem causing physical symptoms. However, stress and tension may add to the pain and increase its intensity.

Do many women have dysmenorrhea?

Yes. Dysmenorrhea is the most common cause of missed work and school hours for women in the United States. It is found most often in women between the ages of 15 and 25.

What causes dysmenorrhea?

For a very small number of women, dysmenorrhea is caused by a disease or physical abnormality. These conditions, such as endometriosis, can be diagnosed and treated.

For most women, dysmenorrhea is not caused by a disease or abnormality. However, it's still not clear exactly what does cause it. The latest research indicates that a group of chemicals produced by your body, called prostaglandins, may cause most of the discomfort.

How could prostaglandins cause dysmenorrhea?

Prostaglandins are responsible for controlling many functions in your body, some of which are linked to dysmenorrhea.

Cramping: Contractions (muscular movements) of your uterus help shed its lining and are controlled by prostaglandins. If greater than normal amounts of prostaglandins are produced, your contractions may be stronger, causing pain in your lower abdomen, back, and thighs.

Headaches, Dizziness: Prostaglandin can constrict ("squeeze") blood vessels. This constriction of blood vessels often leads to an aching head and/or feelings of faintness and dizziness.

Diarrhea, Nausea: Prostaglandin can constrict your large intestines (also called colon). Your colon is where the last stages of food digestion take place. If your colon is constricted, food may be pushed through more rapidly (causing diarrhea), or you may simply feel ill.

Does dysmenorrhea cause serious health problems?

No. Other than the pain and discomfort you feel, dysmenorrhea does not cause serious health problems or make you less able to become pregnant.

Will dysmenorrhea get better over time?

For many women, dysmenorrhea eases or stops as they enter their late twenties and early thirties or have children.

✎ What's It Mean?

Amenorrhea: When a woman does not have periods, either ever (after age 16) or they stop as a result of: pregnancy, too much exercise, extreme obesity or not enough body fat, or emotional distress.

Dysmenorrhea: Painful menstrual periods that can also go along with nausea and vomiting and either constipation or diarrhea. Dysmenorrhea is common among adolescents.

Menstruation: The monthly period or menstrual bleeding. During menstruation, the extra blood and tissue that built up inside the uterus during the menstrual cycle is expelled through the vagina, usually over a period of 3–7 days.

Source: "Girlshealth.gov Web Site Glossary," The National Women's Health Information Center, U.S. Department of Health and Human Services, Office on Women's Health, December 2006.

How can dysmenorrhea be treated?

Listed below are treatment actions you can take:

- Put a heating pad on your abdomen to relax muscles and ease cramping.

- Get adequate sleep and rest.

- Exercise (try walking, swimming, or just dancing to favorite music).

- Do relaxation exercises, such as deep breathing or progressive relaxation.

- Eat a healthy diet.

You may find the following medications helpful: ibuprofen, naproxen sodium (found in Aleve®), birth control pills, prescription medications, calcium-magnesium supplements, and B-complex.

Chapter 24

Premenstrual Syndrome

What is premenstrual syndrome (PMS)?

Premenstrual syndrome (PMS) is a group of symptoms linked to the menstrual cycle. PMS symptoms occur in the week or two weeks before your period (menstruation or monthly bleeding). The symptoms usually go away after your period starts. PMS can affect menstruating women of any age. It is also different for each woman. PMS may be just a monthly bother, or it may be so severe that it makes it hard to even get through the day. Monthly periods stop during menopause, bringing an end to PMS.

What causes PMS?

The causes of PMS are not clear. It is linked to the changing hormones during the menstrual cycle. Some women may be affected more than others by changing hormone levels during the menstrual cycle. Stress and emotional problems do not seem to cause PMS, but they may make it worse.

Diagnosis of PMS is usually based on your symptoms, when they occur, and how much they affect your life.

About This Chapter: The National Women's Health Information Center, U.S. Department of Health and Human Services, Office on Women's Health, January 2007.

What are the symptoms of PMS?

PMS often includes both physical and emotional symptoms. Common symptoms are as follows:

- acne

- breast swelling and tenderness

- feeling tired

- having trouble sleeping

- upset stomach, bloating, constipation, or diarrhea

- headache or backache

- appetite changes or food cravings

- joint or muscle pain

- trouble concentrating or remembering

- tension, irritability, mood swings, or crying spells

- anxiety or depression

> ✔ **Quick Tip**
>
> Symptoms of premenstrual syndrome vary from one woman to another. If you think you have PMS, keep track of which symptoms you have and how severe they are for a few months. You can use a calendar to write down the symptoms you have each day, or you can use a form to track your symptoms. If you go to the doctor for your PMS, take this form with you.

How common is PMS?

Estimates of the percentage of women affected by PMS vary widely. According to the American College of Obstetricians and Gynecologists (ACOG), at least 85 percent of menstruating women have at least one PMS symptom as part of their monthly cycle. Most of these women have symptoms that are fairly mild and do not need treatment. Some women (about three to eight percent of menstruating women) have a more severe form of PMS, called premenstrual dysphoric disorder (PMDD).

PMS occurs more often in women who fall into one or more of these categories:

- are between their late 20s and early 40s

- have at least one child

- have a family history of depression

- have a past medical history of either postpartum depression or a mood disorder

What is the treatment for PMS?

Many things have been tried to ease the symptoms of PMS. No treatment works for every woman, so you may need to try different ones to see what works. If your PMS is not so bad that you need to see a doctor, some lifestyle changes may help you feel better. Below are some lifestyle changes that may help ease your symptoms.

- Take a multivitamin every day that includes 400 micrograms of folic acid. A calcium supplement with vitamin D can help keep bones strong and may help ease some PMS symptoms.

- Exercise regularly.

- Eat healthy foods, including fruits, vegetables, and whole grains.

- Avoid salt, sugary foods, caffeine, and alcohol, especially when you are having PMS symptoms.

- Get enough sleep. Try to get eight hours of sleep each night.

- Find healthy ways to cope with stress. Talk to your friends, exercise, or write in a journal.

- Don't smoke.

Over-the-counter pain relievers, such as ibuprofen, aspirin, or naproxen, may help ease cramps, headaches, backaches, and breast tenderness.

In more severe cases of PMS, prescription medicines may be used to ease symptoms. One approach has been to use drugs such as birth control pills to stop ovulation from occurring. Women on the pill report fewer PMS symptoms, such as cramps and headaches, as well as lighter periods.

What is premenstrual dysphoric disorder (PMDD)?

There is evidence that a brain chemical, called serotonin, plays a role in a severe form of PMS called premenstrual dysphoric disorder (PMDD). The main symptoms, which can be disabling, include the following:

- feelings of sadness or despair, or possibly suicidal thoughts

- feelings of tension or anxiety

- panic attacks

- mood swings, crying

- lasting irritability or anger that affects other people

- disinterest in daily activities and relationships

- trouble thinking or focusing

- tiredness or low energy

- food cravings or binge eating

- having trouble sleeping

- feeling out of control

- physical symptoms, such as bloating, breast tenderness, headaches, and joint or muscle pain

You must have five or more of these symptoms to be diagnosed with PMDD. Symptoms occur during the week before your period and go away after bleeding starts.

Making some lifestyle changes may help ease PMDD symptoms.

Antidepressants, called selective serotonin reuptake inhibitors (SSRIs) that change serotonin levels in the brain, have also been shown to help some women with PMDD. The U.S. Food and Drug Administration (FDA) has approved the following three medications for the treatment of PMDD:

- sertraline (Zoloft®)

- fluoxetine (Sarafem®)

- paroxetine HCI (Paxil CR®)

Individual counseling, group counseling, and stress management may also help relieve symptoms.

Chapter 25

Douching

What is douching?

The word "douche" means to wash or soak in French. Douching is washing or cleaning out the vagina (also called the birth canal) with water or other mixtures of fluids. Usually douches are prepackaged mixes of water and vinegar, baking soda, or iodine. Women can buy these products at drug and grocery stores. The mixtures usually come in a bottle and can be squirted into the vagina through a tube or nozzle.

Why do women douche?

Women douche because they mistakenly believe it gives many benefits. In reality, douching may do more harm than good. Common reasons women give for using douches include the following:

- to clean the vagina
- to rinse away blood after monthly periods
- to get rid of odors from the vagina
- to avoid sexually transmitted diseases (STDs)
- to prevent pregnancy

About This Chapter: The National Women's Health Information Center, U.S. Department of Health and Human Services, Office on Women's Health, December 2005.

How common is douching?

Douching is common among women in the United States. It is estimated that 20 to 40 percent of American women aged 15 to 44 years douche regularly. About half of these women douche every week.

Is douching safe?

Most doctors and the American College of Obstetricians and Gynecologists (ACOG) suggest that women steer clear of douching. All healthy vaginas contain some bacteria and other organisms called the vaginal flora. The normal acidity of the vagina keeps the amount of bacteria down. But douching can change this delicate balance. This may make a woman more prone to vaginal infections. Plus, douching can spread existing vaginal infections up into the uterus, fallopian tubes, and ovaries.

What are the dangers linked to douching?

Research shows that women who douche regularly have more health problems than women who do not. Doctors are still unsure whether douching causes these problems. Douching may simply be more common in groups of women who tend to have these issues. Health problems linked to douching include the following:

- vaginal irritation
- vaginal infections called bacterial vaginosis or BV
- sexually transmitted diseases (STDs)
- pelvic inflammatory disease (PID)

Pelvic inflammatory disease (PID) is an infection of a woman's uterus, fallopian tubes, and/or ovaries. It is caused by bacteria that travel from a woman's vagina and cervix up into her reproductive organs. If left untreated, PID can cause fertility problems (difficulties getting pregnant). PID also boosts a woman's chances of ectopic pregnancy (pregnancy in the fallopian tube instead of the uterus). Some STDs, BV, and PID can all lead to serious problems during pregnancy. These include infection in the baby, problems with labor, and early delivery.

What is the best way to clean my vagina?

Most doctors say that it is best to let your vagina clean itself. The vagina cleans itself naturally by producing mucous. Women do not need to douche to wash away blood, semen, or vaginal discharge. The vagina gets rid of it alone. Also, it is important to note that even healthy, clean vaginas may have a mild odor.

♣ **It's A Fact!!**

Doctors and the American College of Obstetricians and Gynecologists (ACOG) suggest women avoid douching completely. Most experts believe that douching increases a woman's chances of infection. The only time a woman should douche is when her doctor recommends it.

Regular washing with warm water and mild soap during baths and showers will keep the outside of the vagina clean and healthy. Doctors suggest women avoid scented tampons, pads, powders, and sprays. These products may increase a woman's chances of getting vaginal infections.

My vagina has a terrible odor. Can douching help?

No. Douching will only cover up the smell. It will not make it go away. If your vagina has a bad odor, you should call your doctor right away. It could be a sign of a bacterial infection, urinary tract infection, STD, or a more serious problem.

Should I douche to get rid of vaginal discharge, pain, itching, or burning?

No. Douching may even make these problems worse. It is very important to call your doctor right away if you have any of the following:

• vaginal discharge with a bad smell

• thick, white, or yellowish-green discharge with or without a smell

• burning, redness, and swelling of the vagina or the area around it

• pain when urinating

• pain or discomfort during sex

These may be signs of a bacterial infection, yeast infection, urinary tract infection, or STD. Do not douche before seeing your doctor. This can make it hard for the doctor to figure out what is wrong.

Can douching after sex prevent sexually transmitted diseases (STDs)?

No. This is a myth. The only way to completely prevent STDs is to not have sex. But practicing safer sex will dramatically decrease your risk of getting these diseases. You can greatly reduce your chances of getting an STD in the following ways:

- using latex condoms or female condoms every time you have sex
- avoiding contact with sores on the penis or vagina
- preventing the exchange of semen, blood, and vaginal secretions

Can douching after sex stop me from getting pregnant?

No. Douching does not prevent pregnancy and should never be used as a means of birth control. Actually, douching may make it easier to get pregnant by pushing the sperm further up into the vagina and cervix.

Can douching hurt my chances of having a healthy pregnancy?

It may. Limited research shows that douching may make it more difficult for a woman to get pregnant. In women trying to get pregnant, those who douched more than once a week took the longest to get pregnant.

Studies also show that douching may boost a woman's chance of ectopic pregnancy. Ectopic pregnancy is when the fertilized egg attaches to the inside of the fallopian tube instead of the uterus. If left untreated, ectopic pregnancy can be life threatening. It can also make it difficult for a woman to get pregnant in the future.

Chapter 26

First Visit To The Gynecologist

When do I need to go?

A gynecologist is a doctor who has been specially trained in women's reproductive health issues. You should talk to a parent or guardian about seeing a gynecologist (or another doctor who is specially trained in women's health issues) if any of the following is true:

- Have ever had sex (vaginal, oral, or anal) or intimate sexual contact

- Are 21 or older

- Have lower stomach pain, fever, and discharge (fluid coming from your vagina) that is yellow, gray, or green with a strong smell. These may be symptoms of pelvic inflammatory disease (PID). PID is a general term for an infection of the lining of the uterus, fallopian tubes, or the ovaries. Most of the time, PID is caused by sexually transmitted diseases (STDs) such as chlamydia and gonorrhea that have not been treated. Not all vaginal discharges are symptoms of sexually transmitted diseases.

In between periods, it is normal to have a clear or whitish fluid or discharge coming from your vagina. It should not itch or be uncomfortable. It should not smell badly.

About This Chapter: Information in this chapter is from "Do I Need to See a Gynecologist?" GirlsHealth.gov, sponsored by the National Women's Health Information Center, U.S. Department of Health and Human Services, February 2007.

Why do I need to go?

Getting routine gynecology care will do the following:

- Help you understand your body and how it works

- Establish what is normal for you

- Find problems early so they can be treated or kept from getting worse

- Help you understand why it is healthier for you not to have sex while you are a teenager

- Help you learn how to protect yourself if you do have sex

- Help you prepare for healthy relationships and future pregnancies

---

♣ It's A Fact!!

Who Can Care For My Reproductive Health?

- **Your pediatrician.** A pediatrician is a doctor that cares for children and teens. Some pediatricians have special training in reproductive health, but not all. If you are having problems with your period (menstrual cycle), if you think you need to be tested for a sexually transmitted disease, or if you think you may be pregnant, ask your pediatrician. Your pediatrician can help you find someone who can take care of you if you need to see a specialist.

- **A gynecologist.** A gynecologist is a doctor who focuses on women's reproductive health. You may need to visit a gynecologist as you get older.

- **An adolescent specialist.** This type of doctor specializes in caring for teenagers.

- **A nurse practitioner (NP).** A nurse practitioner is a registered nurse with special training. If your clinic or doctor's office has a NP, he or she can do many of the things a doctor can and will work with the doctor if you need special tests or medicines.

- **A family practitioner or general practitioner.** This is a doctor whose practice does not focus on a specific medical specialty, but instead covers varied medical problems in patients of all ages.

Source: Excerpted from "Who Can Care for My Reproductive Health?" GirlsHealth.gov, sponsored by the National Women's Health Information Center, U.S. Department of Health and Human Services, February 2007.

Getting care on a regular basis is important. Your doctor will talk to you about how to take care of your changing body, how to tell if you have a vaginal infection, why abstinence is the healthiest choice, and how to protect yourself from sexually transmitted diseases if you are sexually active. A doctor will also talk to you about your period and will help you out if you are having any problems.

How do I make an appointment?

Talk to your parent or guardian. Or, if you do not think you can talk to your parent or guardian, talk to someone else you trust about how to make an appointment. It is common to feel nervous about going to a clinic, especially when you are a teenager. But being scared is not a reason to skip out. Some of your friends may say they do not need to go, but it is the smart thing to do. A checkup is one important way to keep yourself healthy.

What happens at a visit?

Part of your first visit may be just to talk so you can get to know each other. Your doctor may ask a lot of questions about you and your family. You can also ask the doctor any questions you have. You do not have to be scared or embarrassed. Many teens have the same questions and concerns. You can also talk to your doctor about the following:

- Cramps and problem periods

- Acne

- Weight issues

- Sexually transmitted diseases

- Having the blues or depression

During your visit, your doctor will check your height, weight, and blood pressure. He or she may also do the following exams:

- **Breast Exam:** It is really common for young women to have some lumpiness in their breasts, but your doctor will check your breasts to make sure you do not have strange lumps or pain.

♣ It's A Fact!!
Obstetricians And Gynecologists

What are obstetricians and gynecologists?

Obstetrician-gynecologists specialize in the general medical care of women, as well as care related to pregnancy and the reproductive tract.

What training is required and what is covered?

The obstetrician-gynecologist goes through four years of specialized residency training in areas dealing with preconceptional health, pregnancy, labor and childbirth, postpartum care, genetics, genetic counseling, and prenatal diagnosis.

Training in gynecology also covers women's general health, including care of reproductive organs, breasts, and sexual function.

Screening for cancer at multiple sites is performed or initiated by the Ob-Gyn specialist.

Gynecology also includes management of hormonal disorders, treatment of infections, and training in surgery to correct or treat pelvic organ and urinary tract problems to include cancer of the reproductive organs.

During four years of training, the obstetrician-gynecologist learns about aspects of preventive health care, including exams and routine tests that look for problems before you are sick, immunizations, overall health, and provision of care for a range of medical problems, not just those of the reproductive system.

Source: Reprinted by permission of the American Board of Obstetrics and Gynecology (ABOG). © 2006 American Board of Obstetrics and Gynecology, Inc. All rights reserved. Additional information about certification in obstetrics and gynecology is available at www.abog.org.

- **Pelvic Exam:** The doctor will examine inside your pelvic area to make sure your reproductive organs are healthy. The doctor will check out the outside of your genital area (the vulva) and will then use a tool called a speculum to look inside your vagina to see your cervix. Try to relax and breathe. Finally, the doctor will feel inside to make sure your internal organs feel okay. There will be pressure, but it should not be painful.

- **Pap Test:** If you are 21 or older or within three years of your first sexual experience, you should have a Pap test. This test is done to make sure the cells in your cervix are normal. The doctor will lightly swab your cervix during your pelvic exam to gather cells that can be looked at on a slide at a lab. It is best to have a Pap test when you do not have your period. If there are any problems with your cells, you will be contacted. If you are sexually active, it is especially important to have a Pap test. The Pap test helps the doctor know if more tests are needed to see if you are infected with the human papilloma virus (HPV). Left untreated, this virus can lead to cervical cancer.

Doctors do not always test for sexually transmitted diseases (STDs) during your exam. If you are sexually active, ask to be tested for all STDs.

If it makes you more comfortable, you can have your mom, sister, or a friend stay in the room with you during the exam. If the doctor is male, a female nurse or assistant will also be in the room.

Chapter 27

Pap Test

What is a Pap test?

The Pap test, also called a Pap smear, checks for changes in the cells of your cervix. The cervix is the lower part of the uterus (womb) that opens into the vagina (birth canal). The Pap test can tell if you have an infection, abnormal (unhealthy) cervical cells, or cervical cancer.

Why do I need a Pap test?

A Pap test can save your life. It can find the earliest signs of cervical cancer—a common cancer in women. If caught early, the chance of curing cervical cancer is very high. Pap tests also can find infections and abnormal cervical cells that can turn into cancer cells. Treatment can prevent most cases of cervical cancer from developing.

Do all women need Pap tests?

It is important for all women to have Pap tests, along with pelvic exams, as part of their routine health care. You need a Pap test if you are one of the following:

- 21 years or older

- under 21 years old and have been sexually active for three years or more

About This Chapter: The National Women's Health Information Center, U.S. Department of Health and Human Services, Office on Women's Health, March 2006.

♣ It's A Fact!!
Getting regular Pap tests is the best thing you can do to prevent cervical cancer. In 2004, 3,500 women died from cervical cancer in the United States.

There is no age limit for the Pap test. Even women who have gone through menopause (when a woman's periods stop) need regular Pap tests.

How often do I need to get a Pap test?

It depends on your age and health history. Talk with your doctor about what is best for you. The American College of Obstetricians and Gynecologists recommends the following:

- If you are younger than 30 years old, you should get a Pap test every year.

- If you are age 30 or older and have had three normal Pap tests for three years in a row, talk to your doctor about spacing out Pap tests to every two or three years.

- If you are ages 65 to 70 and have had at least three normal Pap tests and no abnormal Pap tests in the last 10 years, ask your doctor if you can stop having Pap tests.

You should have a Pap test every year no matter how old you are if the following is true:

- You have a weakened immune system because of organ transplant, chemotherapy, or steroid use.

- You are human immunodeficiency virus (HIV) positive.

Women who are living with HIV, the virus that causes acquired immune deficiency syndrome (AIDS), are at a higher risk of cervical cancer and other cervical diseases. The U.S. Centers for Disease Control and Prevention recommends that all HIV positive women get an initial Pap test and get retested six months later. If both Pap tests are normal, then these women can get yearly Pap tests in the future.

Who does not need regular Pap tests?

The only women who do not need regular Pap tests are the following:

- Women over age 65 who have had a number of normal Pap tests and have been told by their doctors that they do not need to be tested anymore.

- Women who do not have a cervix and are at low risk for cervical cancer. These women should speak to their doctor before stopping regular Pap tests.

I had a hysterectomy. Do I still need Pap tests?

It depends on the type of hysterectomy (surgery to remove the uterus) you had and your health history. Women who have had a hysterectomy should talk with their doctor about whether they need routine Pap tests.

Usually during a hysterectomy, the cervix is removed with the uterus. This is called a total hysterectomy. Women who have had a total hysterectomy for reasons other than cancer may not need regular Pap tests. Women who have had a total hysterectomy because of abnormal cells or cancer should be tested yearly for vaginal cancer until they have three normal test results. Women who have had only their uterus removed but still have a cervix need regular Pap tests. Even women who have had hysterectomies should see their doctors yearly for pelvic exams.

How can I reduce my chances of getting cervical cancer?

Aside from getting Pap tests, the best way to avoid cervical cancer is by steering clear of the human papilloma virus (HPV). HPV is a major cause of cervical cancer. HPV infection is also one of the most common sexually transmitted diseases (STDs). So, a woman boosts her chances of getting cervical cancer if she falls into one or more of the following categories:

- Starts having sex before age 18

- Has many sex partners

- Has sex partners who have other sex partners

- Has or has had a sexually transmitted disease (STD)

What should I know about human papilloma viruses (HPV)?

Human papilloma viruses are a group of more than 100 different viruses.

- About 40 types of HPV are spread during sex.

- Some types of HPVs can cause cervical cancer when not treated.

- HPV infection is one of the most common sexually transmitted diseases.

- About 75 percent of sexually active people will get HPV sometime in their life.

- Most women with untreated HPV do not get cervical cancer.

- Some HPVs cause genital warts, but these HPVs do not cause cervical cancer.

- Since HPV rarely causes symptoms, most people do not know they have the infection.

How would I know if I had human papilloma virus (HPV)?

Most women never know they have HPV. It usually stays hidden and does not cause symptoms like warts. When HPV does not go away on its own, it can cause changes in the cells of the cervix. Pap tests usually find these changes.

How do I prepare for a Pap test?

Many things can cause wrong test results by washing away or hiding abnormal cells of the cervix. So, doctors suggest that for two days before the test you avoid the following:

- Douching

- Using tampons

- Using vaginal creams, suppositories, and medicines

- Using vaginal deodorant sprays or powders

- Having sex

> ✔ **Quick Tip**
> Doctors suggest you schedule a Pap test when you do not have your period. The best time to be tested is 10 to 20 days after the first day of your last period.

How is a Pap test done?

Your doctor can do a Pap test during a pelvic exam. It is a simple and quick test. While you lie on an exam table, the doctor puts an instrument called a speculum into your vagina, opening it to see the cervix. She will then use a special stick or brush to take a few cells from inside and around the cervix. The cells are placed on a glass slide and sent to a lab for examination. While usually painless, a Pap test is uncomfortable for some women.

When will I get the results of my Pap test?

Usually it takes three weeks to get Pap test results. Most of the time, test results are normal. If the test shows that something might be wrong, your doctor will contact you to schedule more tests. There are many reasons for abnormal Pap test results. It usually does not mean you have cancer.

What do abnormal Pap test results mean?

It is scary to hear that your Pap test results are abnormal. But abnormal Pap test results usually do not mean you have cancer. Most often there is a small problem with the cervix.

Some abnormal cells will turn into cancer; but most of the time, these unhealthy cells will go away on their own. By treating these unhealthy cells, almost all cases of cervical cancer can be prevented. If you have abnormal results, talk with your doctor about what they mean.

My Pap test was abnormal. What happens now?

There are many reasons for abnormal Pap test results. If results of the Pap test are unclear or show a small change in the cells of the cervix, your doctor will probably repeat the Pap test.

If the test finds more serious changes in the cells of the cervix, the doctor will suggest more powerful tests. Results of these tests will help your doctor decide on the best treatment. These include the following:

- **Colposcopy:** The doctor uses a tool called a colposcope to see the cells of the vagina and cervix in detail.

- **Endocervical Curettage:** The doctor takes a sample of cells from the endocervical canal with a small spoon-shaped tool called a curette.

- **Biopsy:** The doctor removes a small sample of cervical tissue. The sample is sent to a lab to be studied under a microscope.

The FDA recently approved the LUMA Cervical Imaging System. The doctor uses this device right after a colposcopy. This system can help doctors see areas on the cervix that are likely to contain precancerous cells. The doctor uses this device right after a colposcopy. This system shines a light on the cervix and looks at how different areas of the cervix respond to this light. It gives a score to tiny areas of the cervix. It then makes a color map that helps the doctor decide where to further test the tissue with a biopsy. The colors and patterns on the map help the doctor tell between healthy tissue and tissue that might be diseased.

My Pap test result was a false positive. What does this mean?

Pap tests are not always 100 percent correct. False positive and false negative results can happen. This can be upsetting and confusing. A false positive Pap test is when a woman is told she has abnormal cervical cells, but the cells are really normal. If your doctor says your Pap results were a false positive, there is no problem.

A false negative Pap test is when a woman is told her cells are normal, but in fact, there is a problem with the cervical cells that was missed. False negatives delay the discovery and treatment of unhealthy cells of the cervix, but having regular Pap tests boosts your chances of finding any problems. If abnormal cells are missed at one time, they will probably be found on your next Pap test.

Chapter 28

Breast Self-Exam

Breast self-examination can be a useful tool in screening for breast cancer.

The way breasts look and feel is different for every woman. The goal of breast self-examination (BSE) is to become familiar with the way your breasts look and feel to you. Then, if anything changes, you are more likely to notice it earlier so you can see your doctor or nurse as soon as possible.

You can talk to your doctor or nurse about the benefits and limitations of BSE.

If you decide that BSE is right for you, this chapter will help you know how to do it right.

The Three Breast Cancer Screening Tests

Clinical Breast Examination By A Doctor Or Nurse

- Age 20–40: Every three years
- Age 40 and older: Yearly

Mammogram

- Age 40 and older: Yearly

About This Chapter: Reprinted with permission from the State of California Department of Health, Cancer Detection Section brochure, *Breast Self-Examination: Do It For Yourself*, July 2006. © 2006 State of California. All rights reserved.

✔ **Quick Tip**
Some Important Tips To Remember

- Examine your breasts once a month when they are least tender (usually five to ten days from the first day of your period).

- If you no longer have periods, pick another day each month that will remind you to do BSE.

- If you are breastfeeding, empty your breasts first.

- Call your doctor or nurse if anything changes.

Breast Self-Examination

- Age 20 and older: Once a month

Follow The Seven "Ps" Of BSE

Positions (Stand And Lie Down)

Stand to look at your breasts. Standing in front of a mirror, in each of three positions, look for changes in size and shape of the breasts, color and texture of the nipples and skin, and direction your nipples point. Take notice of any staining on your nightclothes or bra from your nipples, especially if only on one side. If things change/look different you should call your doctor or nurse right away.

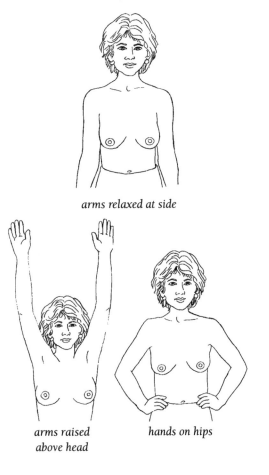

arms relaxed at side

arms raised above head

hands on hips

Figure 28.1. Standing Positions.

Lie down to feel your breasts. Use your left hand to palpate the right breast and your right hand to palpate the left.

Side-Lying Position: Lie on the opposite side of the breast to be examined with your shoulder and hip facing the wall. Rotate just the shoulder (on the same side as the breast to be examined) back to the flat surface. Put the back of your hand on your forehead. Use this position to examine the outer half of your breast to the nipple.

Flat position: When you get to the nipple, lie flat on your back with your arm at a 90° angle to examine the other half of the breast.

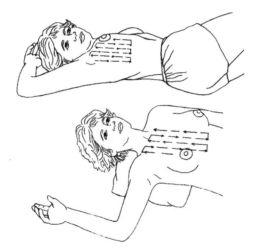

Figure 28.2. Lying Positions: side (top); flat (bottom).

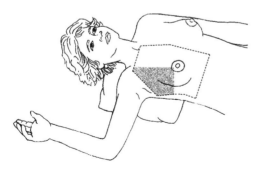

Figure 28.3. Perimeter.

Perimeter (Where To Feel)

The exam area has five sides starting in your armpit down the imaginary seam of your blouse, across your bra line, up your breastbone, across your collarbone, and back to your armpit. Most breast cancers are found in the upper outer area of the breast.

Palpation With Pads Of Fingers (How to Feel)

Use the pads of your three middle fingers together to examine every inch of your breast tissue. Move your fingers in circles about the size of a dime. Do not lift your fingers from your breast between palpations. You can use powder to help your fingers slide from one spot to the next.

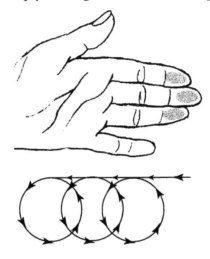

Figure 28.4. Palpation.

Pressure (How Deep To Feel)

Use three levels of pressure for each palpation, from light to deep, to examine the full thickness of your breast tissue. Using pressure is important because the breast is not flat. You need to feel all the way through the tissue to your ribs.

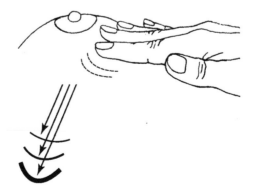

Figure 28.5. Pressure.

Pattern Of Search

Go up and down in rows in the exam area (like mowing a lawn) to examine all of your breast tissue. Be sure to palpate carefully right over the nipple. Start in the armpit and move down to the bra line. Move a finger pad width over and go all the way up to the collarbone. Move a finger pad width over and go back down to the bra line. Keep making these rows until you get to the breastbone. You may need between 12–26 rows to cover all of your breast area. Women who have had breast surgery should also examine the entire area and along the scar.

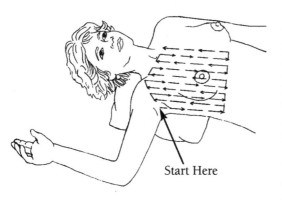

Figure 28.6. Pattern of Search.

Start Here

Practice With Feedback

Have your doctor or nurse show you how to do BSE. Then ask them to watch you do the exam to see that you are doing it right. Ask them to describe and let you feel the different types of tissue in your breast so you know what is normal for you.

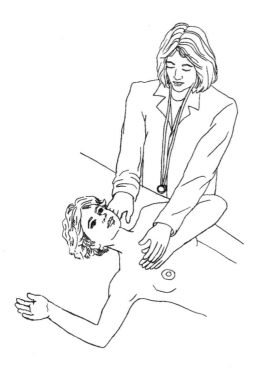

Figure 28.7. Feedback.

Plan Of Action

You should have a personal breast health plan.

Remember!!
If you feel anything new in your breast, call your doctor or nurse right away.

- **Discuss** breast cancer early detection guidelines with your doctor or nurse.

- **Schedule** your clinical breast exam and mammogram as appropriate for your age.

- **Perform** BSE monthly, if you choose to do so.

- **Report** any breast changes to your doctor or nurse.

Chapter 29

Facts About Breast Cancer

The Breasts

The breasts sit on the chest muscles that cover the ribs. Each breast is made of 15 to 20 lobes. Lobes contain many smaller lobules. Lobules contain groups of tiny glands that can produce milk. Milk flows from the lobules through thin tubes called ducts to the nipple. The nipple is in the center of a dark area of skin called the areola. Fat fills the spaces between the lobules and ducts.

The breasts also contain lymph vessels. These vessels lead to small, round organs called lymph nodes. Groups of lymph nodes are near the breast in the axilla (underarm), above the collarbone, in the chest behind the breastbone, and in many other parts of the body. The lymph nodes trap bacteria, cancer cells, or other harmful substances.

Understanding Cancer

Cancer begins in cells, the building blocks that make up tissues. Tissues make up the organs of the body.

Normally, cells grow and divide to form new cells as the body needs them. When cells grow old, they die, and new cells take their place.

About This Chapter: Information in this chapter is from "What You Need To Know About Breast Cancer," National Cancer Institute, U.S. National Institutes of Health, July 2005.

Sometimes, this orderly process goes wrong. New cells form when the body does not need them, and old cells do not die when they should. These extra cells can form a mass of tissue called a growth or tumor.

Tumors can be benign or malignant.

- **Benign tumors** are not cancer.

    - Benign tumors are rarely life threatening.

    - Generally, benign tumors can be removed. They usually do not grow back.

    - Cells from benign tumors do not invade the tissues around them.

    - Cells from benign tumors do not spread to other parts of the body.

- **Malignant tumors** are cancer.

    - Malignant tumors are generally more serious than benign tumors. They may be life threatening.

    - Malignant tumors often can be removed. But sometimes they grow back.

    - Cells from malignant tumors can invade and damage nearby tissues and organs.

    - Cells from malignant tumors can spread (metastasize) to other parts of the body. Cancer cells spread by breaking away from the original (primary) tumor and entering the bloodstream or lymphatic system. The cells invade other organs and form new tumors that damage these organs. The spread of cancer is called metastasis.

When breast cancer cells spread, the cancer cells are often found in lymph nodes near the breast. Also, breast cancer can spread to almost any other part of the body. The most common are the bones, liver, lungs, and brain. The new tumor has the same kind of abnormal cells and the same name as the primary tumor. For example, if breast cancer spreads to the bones, the cancer cells in the bones are actually breast cancer cells. The disease is metastatic breast cancer, not bone cancer. For that reason, it is treated as breast cancer, not bone cancer. Doctors call the new tumor "distant" or metastatic disease.

Risk Factors

No one knows the exact causes of breast cancer. Doctors often cannot explain why one woman develops breast cancer and another does not. They do know that bumping, bruising, or touching the breast does not cause cancer. Breast cancer is not contagious. You cannot catch it from another person.

♣ It's A Fact!!
Breast cancer is the most common type of cancer among women in the U.S. (other than skin cancer).

Research has shown that women with certain risk factors are more likely than others to develop breast cancer. A risk factor is something that may increase the chance of developing a disease.

Studies have found the following risk factors for breast cancer:

- **Age:** The chance of getting breast cancer goes up as a woman gets older. Most cases of breast cancer occur in women over 60. This disease is not common before menopause.

- **Personal history of breast cancer:** A woman who had breast cancer in one breast has an increased risk of getting cancer in her other breast.

- **Family history:** A woman's risk of breast cancer is higher if her mother, sister, or daughter had breast cancer. The risk is higher if her family member got breast cancer before age 40. Having other relatives with breast cancer (in either her mother's or father's family) may also increase a woman's risk.

- **Certain breast changes:** Some women have cells in the breast that look abnormal under a microscope. Having certain types of abnormal cells (atypical hyperplasia and lobular carcinoma in situ [LCIS]) increases the risk of breast cancer.

- **Gene changes:** Changes in certain genes increase the risk of breast cancer. These genes include BRCA1, BRCA2, and others. Tests can sometimes show the presence of specific gene changes in families with many women who have had breast cancer. Health care providers may suggest ways to try to reduce the risk of breast cancer or to improve the detection of this disease in women who have these changes in their genes.

- **Reproductive and menstrual history:**
    - The older a woman is when she has her first child, the greater her chance of breast cancer.
    - Women who had their first menstrual period before age 12 are at an increased risk of breast cancer.
    - Women who went through menopause after age 55 are at an increased risk of breast cancer.
    - Women who never had children are at an increased risk of breast cancer.
    - Women who take menopausal hormone therapy with estrogen plus progestin after menopause also appear to have an increased risk of breast cancer.
    - Large, well-designed studies have shown no link between abortion or miscarriage and breast cancer.

- **Race:** Breast cancer is diagnosed more often in white women than Latina, Asian, or African American women.

- **Radiation therapy to the chest:** Women who had radiation therapy to the chest (including breasts) before age 30 are at an increased risk of breast cancer. This includes women treated with radiation for Hodgkin lymphoma. Studies show that the younger a woman was when she received radiation treatment, the higher her risk of breast cancer later in life.

- **Breast density:** Breast tissue may be dense or fatty. Older women whose mammograms (breast x-rays) show more dense tissue are at increased risk of breast cancer.

- **Being overweight or obese after menopause:** The chance of getting breast cancer after menopause is higher in women who are overweight or obese.

- **Lack of physical activity:** Women who are physically inactive throughout life may have an increased risk of breast cancer. Being active may help reduce risk by preventing weight gain and obesity.

- **Drinking alcohol:** Studies suggest that the more alcohol a woman drinks, the greater her risk of breast cancer.

> **♣ It's A Fact!!**
>
> Each year, more than 211,000 American women learn they have breast cancer.

Other possible risk factors are under study. Researchers are studying the effect of diet, physical activity, and genetics on breast cancer risk. They are also studying whether certain substances in the environment can increase the risk of breast cancer.

Many risk factors can be avoided. Others, such as family history, cannot be avoided. Women can help protect themselves by staying away from known risk factors whenever possible.

It is also important to keep in mind that most women who have known risk factors do not get breast cancer. Also, most women with breast cancer do not have a family history of the disease. In fact, except for growing older, most women with breast cancer have no clear risk factors.

If you think you may be at risk, you should discuss this concern with your doctor. Your doctor may be able to suggest ways to reduce your risk and can plan a schedule for checkups.

Chapter 30

Teens And Breast Implants

Breast implant surgery is a growing trend among teenaged women. According to the American Society for Aesthetic Plastic Surgery (ASAPS), women 18 and under accounted for 11,326 breast implant surgeries performed in American women in 2003, compared to 3,872 in 2002.

Despite more than a decade of controversy over their safety, breast implants are more popular than ever among women who want to build upon what nature gave them or who want to restore what disease has taken away. Whatever the reason, opting for breast implants is a personal decision that should be made only after a woman fully understands and accepts the potential risks of the devices and the importance of follow-up evaluations with her doctor.

Breast implants are designed to change the size and shape of the breast (augmentation), to rebuild the breast (reconstruction), and to replace existing implants (revision). There are two primary types of breast implants: saline-filled and silicone gel-filled. Depending on the type of implant, the shell is either pre-filled with a fixed volume of solution or filled through a valve during the surgery to the desired size. Some allow for adjustments of the filler volume after surgery. Breast implants vary in shape, size, and shell texture.

About This Chapter: From *FDA & You*, Issue #4, Fall 2004, U.S. Food and Drug Administration.

At this time, there are two manufacturers with approved saline-filled breast implants. No manufacturer has yet received FDA approval to market a silicone gel-filled breast implant for augmentation.

Health officials worry that teens and their parents may not realize the risks associated with breast implants. They also want to be sure that the teen's body has finished developing, and that they are psychologically ready to handle the outcome of surgery. While every surgical procedure has potential risks, such as infection, bleeding, and scarring, there are risks that are specific to breast implants. Learning about them is key to being properly informed about the procedure.

"I didn't know my breasts were still growing when I signed up for the surgery," admits Kacey Long, who got saline-filled breast implants in July 2001, when she was 19. Prior to her surgery, the college student from Ennis, Texas, was a 34B, the breast size she thought she would be for life.

Teenagers who are dissatisfied with their bodies see breast implants as harmless and, according to Long, a fun thing to do to improve self-image. Following implantation, Long's breast size increased to a 34D. But complications convinced her to have the implants removed a short time later. Three years later, Long's breasts measured 36C, one size larger than before she was implanted, suggesting that her own breasts continued to develop even after the implants were removed.

Many of the changes to the breast that occur with an implant cannot be undone. If a teen chooses to have her implants removed, she may experience dimpling, puckering, wrinkling, or other cosmetic changes. "When you're making a decision that can impact your life at 19," Long advises other young women, "you need to research the subject like you're 50 years old."

Consider these breast implant facts:

- Breast implants will not last a lifetime. Either because of rupture or other complications, you will likely need to have the implants removed.

- Your breast may not be fully developed and could continue to grow larger, even after implant surgery.

- You are likely to need additional doctor visits and operations because of one or more complications over the course of your life.

- You are likely to have the implants removed, with or without replacement, because of one or more complications over the course of your life.

- Many of the changes to your breasts following implantation may be cosmetically undesirable and cannot be undone.

- If you choose to have your implants removed, you may experience unacceptable dimpling, puckering, wrinkling, loss of breast tissue, or other undesirable cosmetic changes of the breasts.

Chapter 31

Toxic Shock Syndrome

What is toxic shock syndrome?

Toxic shock syndrome (TSS) is a rare, often life-threatening illness that develops suddenly after an infection. TSS can quickly affect several different organ systems including the liver, lungs, and kidneys. Since TSS advances quickly, medical help is needed as soon as possible.

What causes TSS?

TSS is caused by an infection from bacteria. There are two bacteria that produce toxins that can cause TSS—one is *Staphylococcus aureus* (SA), and the other is group A *Streptococcus*. Group A streptococcal bacteria is linked with necrotizing fasciitis or flesh-eating disease.

This chapter describes TSS as it relates to infection with *Staphylococcus aureus* (SA) bacteria.

What is *Staphylococcus aureus*?

SA bacteria are found in the nose and/or on the skin of up to 30 per cent of healthy people. Fortunately these bacteria are usually not harmful and only cause mild throat or skin infections.

About This Chapter: "Toxic Shock Syndrome," BC HealthFile Number 04, October 2005. © 2005 Province of British Columbia. All rights reserved. Reprinted with permission.

SA bacteria produce toxins that do not affect most people. In rare cases, people who have not developed immunity to these toxins can have a severe reaction to them when the toxins get into the bloodstream. This results in toxic shock syndrome.

What are the symptoms of TSS?

Symptoms of TSS include flu-like symptoms, which develop quickly and are severe. Symptoms may include: pain at the site of infection, vomiting and diarrhea, signs of shock including low blood pressure and light-headedness, headache, shortness of breath, and sunburn-like rash.

Symptoms usually develop in three to five days in women who are menstruating and using tampons. In general, TSS symptoms can develop as soon as 12 hours after a surgical procedure.

Who is at risk of TSS?

TSS from SA bacterial infection can affect anyone. However, the majority of affected people are younger women and men, 20 to 40 years of age who have not developed the specific antibodies.

Risk factors for TSS include the following:

- Past history of SA toxic shock syndrome.

- Prolonged use of a tampon, especially the super absorbent type.

- Use of contraceptive sponges, diaphragms, or intrauterine devices.

- Irritation and inflammation of the vagina (vaginitis).

- A skin injury, including a wound from surgery, such as nasal surgery. Those who develop an SA wound infection after surgery may be at greater risk of TSS.

- Recent respiratory infections, such as sinusitis, sore throat (pharyngitis), laryngitis, tonsillitis, or pneumonia.

♣ **It's A Fact!!**
Although menstruating women using tampons are at higher risk of TSS, tampons do not cause TSS.

What should I do if I may have TSS?

If you think you have TSS, you should see a doctor right away. If you cannot see a doctor right away, go to the nearest emergency care facility. If you experience any of the symptoms of TSS while using a tampon, remove the tampon and see a doctor right away. Inform the health professional that you were using a tampon when the symptoms started.

What is the treatment for TSS?

TSS from SA bacterial infection is serious. However, when it is identified and treated correctly, it is fatal in only three to six percent of cases.

TSS cannot be treated at home. Hospital care is required for treating TSS infection and related complications caused by TSS, such as shock. Antibiotic drugs are given to kill the bacteria. If the source of infection involves a tampon, diaphragm, or contraceptive sponge, it should be removed as soon as possible.

Can TSS be prevented?

TSS caused by infection not related to tampon use can be prevented by keeping all wounds clean, including wounds from surgery, cuts, scrapes, burns, sores, and animal or insect bites.

TSS related to use of tampons, diaphragms, or contraceptive sponges can be prevented by doing the following:

- Follow the directions on package inserts when using tampons, diaphragms, or contraceptive sponges.
- Wash your hands with soap before inserting or removing a tampon, diaphragm, or contraceptive sponge.
- Change your tampon at least every eight hours, or use tampons for only part of the day.
- Do not leave your diaphragm or contraceptive sponge in for more than 12 to 18 hours.
- Wear tampons and sanitary pads at alternate times. For example, use pads at night and tampons during the day.
- Use tampons with the lowest absorbency that you need. The risk of TSS is higher with super absorbent tampons.

Chapter 32

Urinary Tract Infection

What is a urinary tract infection (UTI)?

A UTI is an infection anywhere in the urinary tract. Your urinary tract includes the organs that collect and store urine and release it from your body. They are the kidneys, ureters, bladder, and urethra.

What causes a UTI?

Usually, a UTI is caused by bacteria that can also live in the digestive tract, in the vagina, or around the urethra, which is at the entrance to the urinary tract. Most often these bacteria enter the urethra and travel to the bladder and kidneys. Usually, your body removes the bacteria, and you have no symptoms. However, some people seem to be prone to infection, including women and older people.

When should I see my doctor?

You should see your doctor if you have any of these signs or symptoms:

- burning feeling when you urinate

- frequent or intense urges to urinate, even when you have little urine to pass

About This Chapter: Information in this chapter is from "What I Need to Know about Urinary Tract Infections," National Kidney and Urologic Diseases Information Clearinghouse (NKUDIC), a service of the National Institute of diabetes and Digestive and Kidney Diseases (NIDDK), National Institutes of Health (NIH), March 2004.

- pain in your back or lower abdomen

- cloudy, dark, bloody, or unusual-smelling urine

- fever or chills

Women are more likely to get UTIs than men are. When men get UTIs, however, they are often

> ✎ **What's It Mean?**
>
> Kidney: Your kidneys collect wastes and extra water from your blood to make urine.
>
> Ureter: The ureters carry the urine from your kidneys to your bladder.
>
> Bladder: Your bladder stores the urine and squeezes it out when full.
>
> Urethra: The urethra carries the urine out of your bladder when you urinate.

serious and hard to treat. UTIs can be especially dangerous for older people and pregnant women, as well as for those with diabetes and those who have difficulty urinating.

What will happen at the doctor's office?

The doctor may ask you how much fluid you drink, and if you have pain or a burning feeling when you urinate, or if you have difficulty urinating. Women may be asked about the type of birth control they use. You will need to urinate into a cup so the urine can be tested. In addition, your doctor may need to take pictures of your kidneys with an x-ray or ultrasound and look into your bladder with an instrument called a cystoscope. A cystoscope is a thin tube with lenses like a microscope. The tube is inserted into the urinary tract through the urethra.

Your urine will be checked under a microscope for bacteria and infection-fighting cells. The doctor may order a urine culture. In this test, bacteria from the urine are allowed to grow in a lab dish so the exact type of bacteria can be seen and the precise type of medicine you need can be chosen.

How are UTIs treated?

Once it is determined that your symptoms have been caused by an infection, your doctor will prescribe an antibiotic. Antibiotics can kill the bacteria causing the infection. The antibiotic prescribed will depend on the type of bacteria found.

For simple infections, you will be given three days of therapy. For more serious infections, you will be given a prescription for seven days or longer. Be sure to follow your instructions carefully and completely. If you have any allergies to drugs, be sure your doctor knows what they are.

Will UTIs come back?

Sometimes. Most healthy women do not have repeat infections. However, about one out of every five women who get a UTI will get another one. Some women get three or more UTIs a year. Men frequently get repeat infections. Anyone who has diabetes or a problem that makes it difficult to urinate may get repeat infections.

If you get repeat infections, talk with your doctor about special treatment plans. Your doctor may refer you to an urologist, a doctor who specializes in urinary problems. Your doctor may have you take antibiotics over a longer period to help prevent repeat infections. Some doctors give patients who get frequent UTIs a supply of antibiotics to be taken at the first sign of infection. Make sure you understand what your doctor tells you about taking the antibiotic and do exactly that.

How can I keep from getting more UTIs?

Changing some of your daily habits may help you avoid UTIs.

- Drink lots of fluid to flush the bacteria from your system. Water is best. Try for six to eight glasses a day.

- Drink cranberry juice or take vitamin C. Both increase the acid in your urine so bacteria cannot grow easily. Cranberry juice also makes your bladder wall slippery, so bacteria cannot stick to it.

- Urinate frequently and go when you first feel the urge. Bacteria can grow when urine stays in the bladder too long.

- Urinate shortly after sex. This can flush away bacteria that might have entered your urethra during sex.

- After using the toilet, always wipe from front to back, especially after a bowel movement.

- Wear cotton underwear and loose fitting clothes so that air can keep the area dry. Avoid tight-fitting jeans and nylon underwear, which trap moisture and can help bacteria grow.

- For women, using a diaphragm or spermicide for birth control can lead to UTIs by increasing bacteria growth. If you have trouble with UTIs, consider modifying your birth control method. Unlubricated condoms or spermicidal condoms increase irritation and help bacteria cause symptoms. Consider switching to lubricated condoms without spermicide or using a nonspermicidal lubricant.

Chapter 33

Vaginal Yeast Infections And Bacterial Vaginosis

Vaginal Yeast Infections

What is a vaginal yeast infection?

A vaginal yeast infection is irritation of the vagina and the area around the vagina, called the vulva. It is caused by an overgrowth of the fungus or yeast *Candida*. Yeast normally live in the vagina in small numbers, but when the bacteria in the vagina become out of balance, too many yeast grow and cause an infection.

What are the signs of a vaginal yeast infection?

The most common symptom of a yeast infection is extreme itchiness in and around the vagina. Other symptoms include the following:

• Burning, redness, and swelling of the vagina and the area around it

• Pain when urinating

• Pain or discomfort during sex

About This Chapter: Information in this chapter is from "Vaginal Yeast Infections," April 2006, and "Bacterial Vaginosis," May 2005, The National Women's Health Information Center, U.S. Department of Health and Human Services, Office on Women's Health.

- A thick, white vaginal discharge that looks like cottage cheese and does not have a bad smell

You may only have a few of these symptoms, and they may be mild or severe.

Should I call my doctor if I think I have a yeast infection?

Yes. You need to see your doctor to know for sure if you have a yeast infection, especially if you have never had one before. The signs of a yeast infection are similar to those of sexually transmitted diseases (STDs) like chlamydia and gonorrhea. So, it is hard to be sure you have a yeast infection and not something more serious.

If you have had vaginal yeast infections in the past, talk to your doctor about using over-the-counter medicines.

How is a vaginal yeast infection diagnosed?

Your doctor will do a pelvic exam to look for swelling and discharge. She may also use a swab to take a sample from the vagina. A quick look under the microscope or a lab test will show if yeast is causing the problem.

Why did I get a yeast infection?

Many things can change the acidity of the vagina and boost your chances of a vaginal yeast infection. These include the following:

- Stress
- Lack of sleep
- Sickness
- Poor diet or extreme intake of sugary foods
- Pregnancy
- Having your period
- Taking birth control pills
- Taking antibiotics
- Taking steroid medicines
- Diseases such as poorly controlled diabetes and human immunodeficiency virus (HIV) infection

♣ **It's A Fact!!**

Vaginal yeast infections are very common. About 75 percent of women have a yeast infection during their lives, and almost half of women have two or more yeast infections.

Source: Excerpted from "Vaginal Yeast Infections," The National Women's Health Information Center.

Can I get a yeast infection from having sex?

Yes, but it is rare. Women usually do not get yeast infections from sex. Instead, a weakened immune system is the most common cause of yeast infections.

How are yeast infections treated?

Yeast infections can be cured with antifungal medicines in the form of creams, tablets, ointments, or suppositories that are inserted into the vagina. These medicines include butoconazole, clotrimazole, miconazole, nystatin, tioconazole, and terconazole. These products can be bought over the counter at the drug store or grocery store. Your doctor can also prescribe you a single dose of oral fluconazole.

Infections that do not respond to these medicines are becoming more common. Using antifungal medicines when you do not really have a yeast infection can boost your risk of getting a hard-to-treat infection in the future.

Is it safe to use over-the-counter medicines for yeast infections?

Yes, but it is important to talk to your doctor first. Always call your doctor before treating yourself for a vaginal yeast infection if the following is true:

- You are pregnant.
- You have never been diagnosed with a yeast infection.
- You are having repeat yeast infections.

Studies show that two thirds of women who buy these products do not really have a yeast infection. Using these medicines incorrectly may lead to a hard-to-treat infection. Plus, treating yourself for a yeast infection when you really have another kind of infection may worsen the problem.

If you decide to use these over-the-counter medicines, be sure to read and follow the directions carefully. Some creams and inserts may weaken condoms and diaphragms.

If I have a yeast infection, does my sexual partner need to be treated?

Not unless he shows signs of a yeast infection. Rarely, men who have sex with women with yeast infections will get an itchy rash on their penis. If this happens, he should see his doctor.

What should I do if I get repeat yeast infections?

Call your doctor. About five percent of women develop four or more vaginal yeast infections in one year. This is called recurrent vulvovaginal candidiasis (RVVC). RVVC is more common in women with diabetes or weakened immune systems. Doctors normally treat this problem with antifungal medicine for up to six months.

How can I avoid getting another yeast infection?

To help prevent vaginal yeast infections, try the following:

- Do not use douches.
- Avoid scented hygiene products like bubble bath, sprays, pads, and tampons.
- Change tampons and pads often during your period.
- Do not wear tight underwear or clothes made of synthetic fibers.
- Wear cotton underwear and pantyhose with a cotton crotch.
- Change out of wet swimsuits and exercise clothes as soon as possible.

If you have repeat yeast infections, talk to your doctor.

Bacterial Vaginosis

What is bacterial vaginosis (BV)?

Bacterial vaginosis, also called BV, is the most common vaginal infection in women of childbearing age. It happens when the normal balance of bacteria in the vagina is disrupted and replaced by an overgrowth of certain bacteria. The vagina normally contains mostly "good" bacteria and fewer "harmful" bacteria. BV develops when there is an increase in "harmful" bacteria and fewer "good" bacteria.

What causes BV?

The cause of BV is not understood. It can develop when something, like sexual contact, disrupts the balance between the good bacteria that protect the vagina from infection and the harmful bacteria that do not. It is not clear what role sexual activity plays in the development of BV, but BV is more common among women who have had vaginal sex. But BV is not always from sexual contact. We do know that certain things can upset the normal balance of bacteria in the vagina and put you more at risk for BV. They are as follows: having a new sex partner or multiple sex partners; douching; using an intrauterine device (IUD) for birth control; not using a condom.

What are the signs of BV?

Women with BV may have an abnormal vaginal discharge with an unpleasant odor. Some women report a strong fish-like odor, especially after sexual intercourse. The discharge can be white (milky) or gray and thin. Other symptoms may include burning when urinating, itching around the outside of the vagina, and irritation. However, these could be symptoms of another infection too. Some women with BV have no symptoms at all.

How can I find out if I have BV?

There is a test to find out if you have BV. Your doctor takes a sample of fluid from your vagina and has it tested. Your doctor may also be able to see signs of BV, like a grayish-white discharge, during an examination of the vagina.

♣ It's A Fact!!
You do not get BV from toilet seats, bedding, swimming pools, or from touching objects around you.

Source: Excerpted from "Bacterial Vaginosis," The National Women's Health Information Center.

How is BV treated?

BV is treated with antibiotics, which are medicines prescribed by your doctor. Your doctor may give you either metronidazole or clindamycin. Generally, male sex partners of women with BV do not need to be treated. You can get BV again even after being treated.

Can BV cause medical problems?

In most cases, BV does not cause any problems. But some problems can happen if BV is untreated. They are as follows:

- **Pregnancy Problems:** BV can cause premature delivery and low birth weight babies (less than five pounds).

- **Pelvic Inflammatory Disease (PID):** PID is an infection that can affect a woman's uterus, ovaries, and fallopian tubes, which carry eggs from the ovaries to the uterus. Having BV increases the risk of getting PID after a surgical procedure, such as a hysterectomy or an abortion.

- **Higher Risk of Getting Other STDs:** Having BV can increase the chances of getting other STDs, such as chlamydia, gonorrhea, and HIV. Women with HIV who get BV increase the chances of passing HIV to a sexual partner.

How can I prevent BV?

BV is not well understood by scientists, and the best ways to prevent it are unknown. What is known is that BV is associated with having a new sex partner or having multiple sex partners. Follow these tips to lower your risk for getting BV:

- **Do not have sex.** The best way to prevent any STD is to practice abstinence or not having vaginal, oral, or anal sex.

- **Be faithful.** Have a sexual relationship with one partner is another way to reduce your chances of getting infected. Be faithful to each other, meaning that you only have sex with each other and no one else.

- **Use condoms.** Protect yourself with a condom every time you have vaginal, anal, or oral sex. Condoms should be used for any type of sex with every partner. For vaginal sex, use a latex male condom or a female polyurethane condom. For anal sex, use a latex male condom. For oral sex, use a dental dam. A dental dam is a rubbery material that can be placed over the anus or the vagina before sexual contact.

- **Do not douche.** Douching removes some of the normal bacteria in the vagina that protects you from infection. This may increase your chances of getting BV. It may also increase the chances of BV coming back after treatment.

- **Talk with your sex partner(s) about STDs and using condoms.** It is up to you to make sure you are protected. Remember, it is your body.

- **Talk frankly with your doctor or nurse and your sex partner(s) about any STDs you or your partner have or had.** Talk about any discharge in the genital area. Try not to be embarrassed.

- **Have regular pelvic exams.** Talk with your doctor about how often you need them. Many tests for STDs can be done during an exam.

- **If you are pregnant and have symptoms of BV, or had a premature delivery or low birth weight baby in the past, get tested for BV.** Get tested as soon as you think you may be pregnant.

- **Finish your medicine.** If you have BV, finish all the medicine that you are given to treat it. Even if the symptoms go away, you still need to finish all of the medicine.

Chapter 34

Pelvic Inflammatory Disease

What is pelvic inflammatory disease (PID)?

Pelvic inflammatory disease (PID) is a general term that refers to infection of the uterus (womb), fallopian tubes (tubes that carry eggs from the ovaries to the uterus), and other reproductive organs. It is a common and serious complication of some sexually transmitted diseases (STDs), especially chlamydia and gonorrhea. PID can damage the fallopian tubes and tissues in and near the uterus and ovaries. Untreated PID can lead to serious consequences including infertility, ectopic pregnancy (a pregnancy in the fallopian tube or elsewhere outside of the womb), abscess formation, and chronic pelvic pain.

How common is PID?

Each year in the United States, it is estimated that more than one million women experience an episode of acute PID. More than 100,000 women become infertile each year as a result of PID, and a large proportion of the ectopic pregnancies occurring every year are due to the consequences of PID. Annually more than 150 women die from PID or its complications.

About This Chapter: Information in this chapter is from "Pelvic Inflammatory Disease—CDC Fact Sheet," Centers for Disease Control and Prevention, U.S. Department of Health and Human Services, May 2004.

How do women get PID?

PID occurs when bacteria move upward from a woman's vagina or cervix (opening to the uterus) into her reproductive organs. Many different organisms can cause PID, but many cases are associated with gonorrhea and chlamydia, two very common bacterial STDs. A prior episode of PID increases the risk of another episode because the reproductive organs may be damaged during the initial bout of infection.

> ### ♣ It's A Fact!!
>
> Sexually active women in their childbearing years are most at risk, and those under age 25 are more likely to develop pelvic inflammatory disease (PID) than those older than 25. This is because the cervix of teenage girls and young women is not fully matured, increasing their susceptibility to the sexually transmitted diseases (STDs) that are linked to PID.

The more sex partners a woman has, the greater her risk of developing PID. Also, a woman whose partner has more than one sex partner is at greater risk of developing PID because of the potential for more exposure to infectious agents.

Women who douche may have a higher risk of developing PID compared with women who do not douche. Research has shown that douching changes the vaginal flora (organisms that live in the vagina) in harmful ways and can force bacteria into the upper reproductive organs from the vagina.

Women who have an intrauterine device (IUD) inserted may have a slightly increased risk of PID near the time of insertion compared with women using other contraceptives or no contraceptive at all. However, this risk is greatly reduced if a woman is tested and, if necessary, treated for STDs before an IUD is inserted.

What are the signs and symptoms of PID?

Symptoms of PID vary from none to severe. When PID is caused by chlamydial infection, a woman may experience mild symptoms or no symptoms at all, while serious damage is being done to her reproductive organs. Because of vague symptoms, PID goes unrecognized by women and their health care providers about two thirds of the time. Women who have symptoms of

PID most commonly have lower abdominal pain. Other signs and symptoms include fever, unusual vaginal discharge that may have a foul odor, painful intercourse, painful urination, irregular menstrual bleeding, and pain in the right upper abdomen (rare).

What are the complications of PID?

Prompt and appropriate treatment can help prevent complications of PID. Without treatment, PID can cause permanent damage to the female reproductive organs. Infection-causing bacteria can silently invade the fallopian tubes, causing normal tissue to turn into scar tissue. This scar tissue blocks or interrupts the normal movement of eggs into the uterus. If the fallopian tubes are totally blocked by scar tissue, sperm cannot fertilize an egg, and the woman becomes infertile. Infertility also can occur if the fallopian tubes are partially blocked or even slightly damaged. About one in eight women with PID becomes infertile; and if a woman has multiple episodes of PID, her chances of becoming infertile increase.

In addition, a partially blocked or slightly damaged fallopian tube may cause a fertilized egg to remain in the fallopian tube. If this fertilized egg begins to grow in the tube as if it were in the uterus, it is called an ectopic pregnancy. As it grows, an ectopic pregnancy can rupture the fallopian tube causing severe pain, internal bleeding, and even death.

Scarring in the fallopian tubes and other pelvic structures can also cause chronic pelvic pain (pain that lasts for months or even years). Women with repeated episodes of PID are more likely to suffer infertility, ectopic pregnancy, or chronic pelvic pain.

How is PID diagnosed?

PID is difficult to diagnose because the symptoms are often subtle and mild. Many episodes of PID go undetected because the woman or her health care provider fails to recognize the implications of mild or nonspecific symptoms. Because there are no precise tests for PID, a diagnosis is usually based on clinical findings. If symptoms such as lower abdominal pain are present, a health care provider should perform a physical examination to determine the nature and location of the pain and check for fever, abnormal vaginal or cervical discharge, and for evidence of gonorrheal or chlamydial infection. If the findings suggest PID, treatment is necessary.

The health care provider may also order tests to identify the infection-causing organism (for example, chlamydial or gonorrheal infection) or to distinguish between PID and other problems with similar symptoms. A pelvic ultrasound is a helpful procedure for diagnosing PID. An ultrasound can view the pelvic area to see whether the fallopian tubes are enlarged or whether an abscess is present. In some cases, a laparoscopy may be necessary to confirm the diagnosis. A laparoscopy is a minor surgical procedure in which a thin, flexible tube with a lighted end (laparoscope) is inserted through a small incision in the lower abdomen. This procedure enables the doctor to view the internal pelvic organs and to take specimens for laboratory studies, if needed.

What is the treatment for PID?

PID can be cured with several types of antibiotics. A health care provider will determine and prescribe the best therapy. However, antibiotic treatment does not reverse any damage that has already occurred to the reproductive organs. If a woman has pelvic pain and other symptoms of PID, it is critical that she seek care immediately. Prompt antibiotic treatment can prevent severe damage to reproductive organs. The longer a woman delays treatment for PID, the more likely she is to become infertile or to have a future ectopic pregnancy because of damage to the fallopian tubes.

Because of the difficulty in identifying organisms infecting the internal reproductive organs and because more than one organism may be responsible for an episode of PID, PID is usually treated with at least two antibiotics that are effective against a wide range of infectious agents. These antibiotics can be given by mouth or by injection. The symptoms may go away before the infection is cured. Even if symptoms go away, the woman should finish taking all of the prescribed medicine. This will help prevent the infection from returning. Women being treated for PID should be re-evaluated by their health care provider two to three days after starting treatment to be sure the antibiotics are working to cure the infection. In addition, a woman's sex partner(s) should be treated to decrease the risk of re-infection, even if the partner(s) has no symptoms. Although sex partners may have no symptoms, they may still be infected with the organisms that can cause PID.

Hospitalization to treat PID may be recommended if the woman is severely ill (for example, nausea, vomiting, and high fever); is pregnant; does not respond to, or cannot take oral medication, and needs intravenous antibiotics; or has an abscess in the fallopian tube or ovary (tubo-ovarian abscess). If symptoms continue, or if an abscess does not go away, surgery may be needed. Complications of PID, such as chronic pelvic pain and scarring are difficult to treat, but sometimes they improve with surgery.

How can PID be prevented?

Women can protect themselves from PID by taking action to prevent STDs or by getting early treatment if they do get an STD.

♣ It's A Fact!!

Sexually transmitted disease (STD), mainly untreated chlamydia or gonorrhea, is the main preventable cause of pelvic inflammatory disease (PID).

The surest way to avoid transmission of STDs is to abstain from sexual intercourse or to be in a long-term mutually monogamous relationship with a partner who has been tested and is known to be uninfected.

Latex male condoms, when used consistently and correctly, can reduce the risk of transmission of chlamydia and gonorrhea.

Centers for Disease Control and Prevention (CDC) recommends yearly chlamydia testing of all sexually active women age 25 or younger and of older women with risk factors for chlamydial infections (those who have a new sex partner or multiple sex partners). An appropriate sexual risk assessment by a health care provider should always be conducted and may indicate more frequent screening for some women.

Any genital symptoms such as an unusual sore, discharge with odor, burning during urination, or bleeding between menstrual cycles could mean an STD infection. If a woman has any of these symptoms, she should stop having sex and consult a health care provider immediately. Treating STDs early can prevent PID. Women who are told they have an STD and are treated for it should notify all of their recent sex partners so they can see a health care provider and be evaluated for STDs. Sexual activity should not resume until all sex partners have been examined and, if necessary, treated.

Chapter 35

Endometriosis

What is endometriosis?

Endometriosis is a common health problem in women. It gets its name from the word endometrium, the tissue that lines the uterus (womb). In women with this problem, tissue that looks and acts like the lining of the uterus grows outside of the uterus in other areas. These areas can be called growths, tumors, implants, lesions, or nodules.

Most endometriosis is found in these areas:

- on or under the ovaries
- behind the uterus
- on the tissues that hold the uterus in place
- on the bowels or bladder

Endometriosis rarely grows in the lungs or other parts of the body. This "misplaced" tissue can cause pain, infertility (not being able to get pregnant), and very heavy periods.

What are the symptoms of endometriosis?

Pain is one of the most common symptoms of endometriosis. Usually the pain is in the abdomen, lower back, and pelvis. The amount of pain a woman

About This Chapter: The National Women's Health Information Center, U.S. Department of Health and Human Services, Office on Women's Health, July 2006.

feels does not depend on how much endometriosis she has. Some women have no pain, even though their disease affects large areas. Other women with endometriosis have severe pain even though they have only a few small growths. Symptoms of endometriosis include the following:

- very painful menstrual cramps

- pain with periods that gets worse over time

- chronic pain in the lower back and pelvis

- pain during or after sex

- intestinal pain

- painful bowel movements or painful urination during menstrual periods

- heavy and/or long menstrual periods

- spotting or bleeding between periods

- infertility (not being able to get pregnant)

- fatigue

♣ It's A Fact!!
About five million women in the United States have endometriosis. This makes it one of the most common health problems for women.

Women with endometriosis may also have gastrointestinal problems such as diarrhea, constipation, or bloating, especially during their periods.

Who usually gets endometriosis?

In general, women with endometriosis meet the following criteria:

- get their monthly period

- are 27 years old on average

- have symptoms for two to five years before finding out they have the disease

Women who have gone through menopause (when a woman stops having her period) rarely still have symptoms.

What can raise my chances of getting endometriosis?

You are more likely to develop endometriosis if you meet the following criteria:

- began getting your period at an early age
- have heavy periods
- have periods that last more than seven days
- have a short monthly cycle (27 days or less)
- have a close relative (mother, aunt, sister) with endometriosis

How can I reduce my chances of getting endometriosis?

Some studies suggest that you may lower your chances of developing endometriosis if you do the following:

- exercise regularly
- avoid alcohol and caffeine

Why do patches of endometriosis cause pain and health problems?

Growths of endometriosis are almost always benign or not cancerous but still can cause many problems. To see why, it helps to understand a woman's monthly cycle. Every month, hormones cause the lining of a woman's uterus to build up with tissue and blood vessels. If a woman does not get pregnant, the uterus sheds this tissue and blood. It comes out of the body through the vagina as her menstrual period.

Patches of endometriosis also respond to a woman's monthly cycle. Each month the growths add extra tissue and blood, but there is no place for the built-up tissue and blood to exit the body. For this reason, growths tend to get bigger, and the symptoms of endometriosis often get worse over time.

Tissue and blood that is shed into the body can cause inflammation, scar tissue, and pain. As the misplaced tissue grows, it can cover or grow into the ovaries and block the fallopian tubes. This can make it hard for women with endometriosis to get pregnant. The growths can also cause problems in the intestines and bladder.

Why is it important to find out if I have endometriosis?

The pain of endometriosis can interfere with your life. Studies show that women with endometriosis often skip school, work, and social events. This health problem can also get in the way of relationships with your partner, friends, and co-workers. Plus, endometriosis can make it hard for you to get pregnant when you are ready.

Finding out that you have endometriosis is the first step in taking back your life. Many treatments can control the symptoms. Medicine can relieve your pain; and when endometriosis causes fertility problems, surgery can boost your chances of getting pregnant.

How would I know if I have endometriosis?

If you think you have this disease, talk with your obstetrician/gynecologist (OB/GYN). Your OB/GYN has special training to diagnose and treat this condition. The doctor will talk to you about your symptoms and health history. Then she or he will do a pelvic exam. Sometimes during the exam, the doctor can find signs of endometriosis.

Usually doctors need to run tests to find out if a woman has endometriosis. Sometimes doctors use imaging tests to "see" large growths of endometriosis inside the body. The two most common imaging tests are the following:

- ultrasound, which uses sound waves to see inside the body

- magnetic imaging (MRI), which uses magnets and radio waves to make a "picture" of the inside of the body

The only way to know for sure if you have endometriosis is to have a surgery called laparoscopy. In this procedure, a tiny cut is made in your abdomen. A thin tube with a light is placed inside to see growths from endometriosis. Sometimes doctors can diagnose endometriosis just by seeing the growths. Other times, they need to take a small sample of tissue, or a biopsy, and study it under a microscope.

What causes endometriosis?

No one knows for sure what causes this disease, but scientists have a number of theories. They know that endometriosis runs in families. So, one theory suggests that endometriosis is caused by genes.

Another theory is that during a woman's monthly periods, some endometrial tissue backs up into the abdomen through the fallopian tubes. This transplanted

♣ It's A Fact!!

If your mother or sister has endometriosis, you are six times more likely to get the disease than other women.

tissue then grows outside the uterus. Many researchers think a faulty immune system plays a part in endometriosis. In women with the disease, the immune system fails to find and destroy endometrial tissue growing outside of the uterus. Plus, a recent study shows that immune system disorders (health problems in which the body attacks itself) are more common in women with endometriosis. More research in this area may help doctors better understand and treat endometriosis.

How is endometriosis treated?

There is no cure for endometriosis, but there are many treatments for the pain and infertility that it causes. Talk with your doctor about what option is best for you. The treatment you choose will depend on your symptoms, age, and plans for getting pregnant.

Pain Medication: For some women with mild symptoms, doctors may suggest taking over-the-counter medicines for pain. These include: ibuprofen (Advil and Motrin) or naproxen (Aleve). When these medicines do not help, doctors may advise using stronger pain relievers available by prescription.

Hormone Treatment: When pain medicine is not enough, doctors often recommend hormone medicines to treat endometriosis. Only women who do not wish to become pregnant can use these drugs. Hormone treatment is best for women with small growths who do not have bad pain.

Hormones come in many forms including pills, shots, and nasal sprays.

Surgery: Surgery is usually the best choice for women with endometriosis who have a severe amount of growths, a great deal of pain, or fertility problems. There are both minor and more complex surgeries that can help. Your doctor might suggest one of the following:

- *Laparoscopy* can be used to diagnose and treat endometriosis. During this surgery, doctors remove growths and scar tissue or destroy them with intense heat. The goal is to treat the endometriosis without harming the healthy tissue around it. Women recover from laparoscopy much faster than from major abdominal surgery.

- *Laparotomy or major abdominal surgery* is a last resort treatment for severe endometriosis. In this surgery, the doctor makes a much bigger cut in the abdomen than with laparoscopy. This allows the doctor to reach and remove growths of endometriosis in the pelvis or abdomen. Recovery from this surgery can take up to two months.

- *Hysterectomy* should only be considered by women who do not want to become pregnant in the future. During this surgery, the doctor removes the uterus. She or he may also take out the ovaries and fallopian tubes at the same time. This is done when the endometriosis has severely damaged them.

How do I cope with a disease that has no cure?

You may feel many emotions—sadness, fright, anger, confusion, and loneliness. It is important to get support to cope with endometriosis. Consider joining a support group to talk with other women who have endometriosis. There are support groups on the internet and in many communities.

It is also important to learn as much as you can about the disease. Talking with friends, family, and your doctor can help.

Chapter 36

Turner Syndrome

Turner syndrome affects approximately 1 out of every 2,500 female live births worldwide. It embraces a broad spectrum of features, from major heart defects to minor cosmetic issues. Some individuals with Turner syndrome may have only a few features, while others may have many. Almost all people with Turner syndrome have short stature and loss of ovarian function, but the severity of these problems varies considerably amongst individuals.

Appearance

Individuals with Turner syndrome may have a short neck with a webbed appearance, a low hairline at the back of the neck, and low-set ears. Hands and feet of affected individuals may be swollen or puffy at birth and often have soft nails that turn upward at the ends when they are older. All these features appear to be due to obstruction of the lymphatic system during fetal development. Another characteristic cosmetic feature is the presence of multiple pigmented nevi, which are colored spots on the skin.

Short Stature

Almost all individuals with Turner syndrome have short stature. This is partially due to the loss of action SHOX gene on the X-chromosome. This particular

About This Chapter: Information in this chapter is from "Clinical Features of Turner Syndrome," National Institute of Child Health and Human Development, National Institutes of Health, September 2004.

gene is important for long bone growth. The loss of SHOX may also explain some of the skeletal features found in Turner syndrome, such as short fingers and toes, and irregular rotations of the wrist and elbow joints. Growth lags during childhood and adolescence, resulting in adult heights of approximately 4 feet 8 inches. Final adult height in Turner syndrome can be increased by a few inches if growth hormone (GH) treatment is given relatively early in childhood. However, not all individuals with Turner syndrome get a good growth response to GH.

Puberty And Reproduction

Unknown genes on the X-chromosome regulate the development and functions of the ovary.

Some teenagers may undergo some breast development and begin menstruating but cease further development and menses during the later teen years. A few women with Turner syndrome have apparently normal ovarian function with regular menses until the mid-20s before ovarian failure occurs. A few spontaneous pregnancies have been reported.

> ♣ **It's A Fact!!**
> Most individuals with Turner syndrome experience loss of ovarian function early in childhood, and thus do not enter puberty at the normal age.

It is standard medical practice to treat girls with Turner syndrome with estrogen to induce breast development and other features of puberty if menses has not occurred by age 15 years at the latest. Girls and women with Turner syndrome should be maintained on estrogen-progesterone treatment to maintain their secondary sexual development and to protect their bones from osteoporosis until at least the usual age of menopause (50 years).

Most women with Turner syndrome do not have ovaries with healthy oocytes capable of fertilization and embryo formation. Current assisted reproductive technology, however, may allow women to become pregnant with donated oocytes.

Cardiovascular

From 5–10% of children with Turner syndrome are found to have a severe constriction of the major blood vessel coming out from the heart, a condition known as "coarctation of the aorta." This defect is thought to be the result of an obstructed lymphatic system compressing the developing aorta during fetal life. This can be surgically corrected as soon as it is diagnosed.

Other major defects in the heart and its major vessels are reported to a much lesser degree. As many as 15% of adults with Turner syndrome are reported to have "bicuspid aortic valves," meaning that the major blood vessel from the heart has only two rather than three components to the valve regulating blood flow. This condition has been discovered mainly by medical imaging studies on women without symptoms and may not be clinically obvious. It requires careful medical monitoring, since bicuspid aortic valves can deteriorate or become infected. In general, it is advised that all persons with Turner syndrome undergo annual cardiac evaluations.

Many women with Turner syndrome have high blood pressure, which may be apparent even in childhood. In some cases this high blood pressure may be due to aortic constriction or to kidney abnormalities. In a majority of women, however, no specific cause for the high blood pressure has been found.

Kidney

Kidney problems are present in approximately one-third of individuals with Turners and may contribute to high blood pressure. Three types of kidney problems have been reported: a single horseshoe-shaped kidney, as opposed to two distinct, bean-shaped structures; an abnormal urine collecting system; or an abnormal artery supply to the kidneys. While these problems may be corrected surgically, and the kidneys usually function normally, they may be associated with a tendency towards high blood pressure and infections.

Osteoporosis

There is a high incidence of osteoporosis, meaning thin or weak bones, in women with Turner syndrome. Osteoporosis leads to loss of height, curvature of the spine, and increased bone fractures.

The primary cause of osteoporosis in individuals with Turners appears to be inadequate circulating estrogen in the body. Turner women who have low levels of estrogen due to ovarian failure can take estrogen treatments, which will help prevent osteoporosis. It is possible that other factors contribute to the severity of osteoporosis in Turner syndrome. For example, there may be defects in bone structure or strength related to the loss of unknown X-chromosome genes. This is an area of major medical significance, which demands further study to help prevent osteoporosis and fractures in women with Turner syndrome.

Diabetes

Type II diabetes, also known as insulin resistant diabetes (glucose intolerance), has a high occurrence rate in individuals with Turner syndrome.

Individuals with Turner syndrome have twice the risk of the general population for developing this disease. It appears that the muscles of many persons with Turner syndrome fail to utilize glucose efficiently, and this may contribute to the development of high blood sugar (diabetes).

The reason for the high risk of diabetes among individuals with Turner syndrome is unknown.

Diabetes type II can be controlled through careful monitoring of blood sugar levels, diet, exercise, regular doctor visits, and sometimes medication.

Thyroid

Approximately one-third of individuals with Turner syndrome have a thyroid disorder, usually hypothyroidism. Symptoms of this condition include decreased energy, dry skin, cold intolerance, and poor growth.

In most cases, it is caused by an immune system attack on the thyroid gland (also known as Hashimoto thyroiditis). Although it is not known why thyroid disorders occur with a high frequency in Turner syndrome, the condition is easily treated with thyroid hormone supplements.

Cognitive Function And Educational Issues

In general, individuals with Turner syndrome have normal intelligence. This is in contrast to other chromosomal syndromes such as Down syndrome (Trisomy 21). However, girls and women with Turner syndrome may have difficulty with specific visual-spatial coordination tasks (for example, mentally rotating objects in space) and learning math (geometry, arithmetic). This very specific learning problem has been termed the "Turner neurocognitive phenotype" and appears due to loss of X-chromosome genes important for selected aspects of nervous system development.

Some girls and women with Turner syndrome experience difficulties with memory and motor coordination. These problems may be related to estrogen deficiency, and individuals often improve when given estrogen treatment. The verbal skills of individuals with Turner syndrome are usually normal.

Part Four

For Guys Only

Chapter 37

The Male Reproductive System:
An Overview

The male reproductive system, like that of the female, consists of those organs whose function is to produce a new individual, i.e., to accomplish reproduction. This system consists of a pair of testes and a network of excretory ducts (epididymis, ductus deferens (vas deferens), and ejaculatory ducts), seminal vesicles, the prostate, the bulbourethral glands, and the penis.

Testes

The male gonads, testes, or testicles, begin their development high in the abdominal cavity, near the kidneys. During the last two months before birth, or shortly after birth, they descend through the inguinal canal into the scrotum, a pouch that extends below the abdomen, posterior to the penis. Although this location of the testes, outside the abdominal cavity, may seem to make them vulnerable to injury, it provides a temperature about 3° C below normal body temperature. This lower temperature is necessary for the production of viable sperm. The scrotum consists of skin and subcutaneous tissue. A vertical septum, or partition, of subcutaneous tissue in the center divides

About This Chapter: Information in this chapter is from "Reproductive System," from the National Cancer Institute's Surveillance, Epidemiology and End Results (SEER) Training Web Site, 2000. Note: Despite the older date of this document, the anatomical information it presents is still current.

it into two parts, each containing one testis. Smooth muscle fibers, called the dartos muscle, in the subcutaneous tissue contract to give the scrotum its wrinkled appearance. When these fibers are relaxed, the scrotum is smooth. Another muscle, the cremaster muscle, consists of skeletal muscle fibers and controls the position of the scrotum and testes. When it is cold or a man is sexually aroused, this muscle contracts to pull the testes closer to the body for warmth.

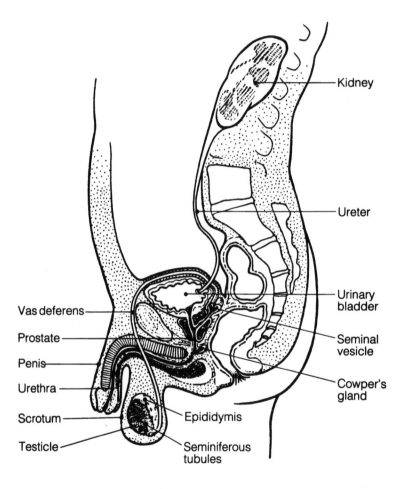

Figure 37.1. Male Reproductive System (Source: Cancer Visuals Online, National Cancer Institute)

Structure

Each testis is an oval structure about 5 cm long and 3 cm in diameter. A tough, white fibrous connective tissue capsule, the tunica albuginea, surrounds each testis and extends inward to form septa that partition the organ into lobules. There are about 250 lobules in each testis. Each lobule contains 1 to 4 highly coiled seminiferous tubules that converge to form a single straight tubule, which leads into the rete testis. Short efferent ducts exit the testes. Interstitial cells (cells of Leydig), which produce male sex hormones, are located between the seminiferous tubules within a lobule.

Spermatogenesis

Sperm are produced by spermatogenesis within the seminiferous tubules. A transverse section of a seminiferous tubule shows that it is packed with cells in various stages of development. Interspersed with these cells, there are large cells that extend from the periphery of the tubule to the lumen. These large cells are the supporting, or sustentacular cells (Sertoli cells), which support and nourish the other cells.

Early in embryonic development, primordial germ cells enter the testes and differentiate into spermatogonia, immature cells that remain dormant until puberty. Spermatogonia are diploid cells, each with 46 chromosomes (23 pairs) located around the periphery of the seminiferous tubules. At puberty, hormones stimulate these cells to begin dividing by mitosis. Some of the daughter cells produced by mitosis remain at the periphery as spermatogonia. Others are pushed toward the lumen, undergo some changes, and become primary spermatocytes. Because they are produced by mitosis, primary spermatocytes, like spermatogonia, are diploid and have 46 chromosomes.

Each primary spermatocyte goes through the first meiotic division, meiosis I, to produce two secondary spermatocytes, each with 23 chromosomes (haploid). Just prior to this division, the genetic material is replicated so that each chromosome consists of two strands, called chromatids, which are joined by a centromere. During meiosis I, one chromosome, consisting of two chromatids, goes to each secondary spermatocyte. In the second meiotic division, meiosis II, each secondary spermatocyte divides to produce two spermatids. There is no replication of genetic material in this division, but the centromere divides so that a single-stranded chromatid goes to each cell. As a result of the two meiotic divisions, each primary spermatocyte produces four spermatids. During spermatogenesis there are two cellular divisions, but only one replication of DNA so that each spermatid has 23 chromosomes (haploid), one from each pair in the original primary spermatocyte. Each successive stage in spermatogenesis is pushed toward the center of the tubule so that the more immature cells are at the periphery and the more differentiated cells are nearer the center.

Spermatogenesis (and oogenesis in the female) differs from mitosis because the resulting cells have only half the number of chromosomes as the original cell. When the sperm cell nucleus unites with an egg cell nucleus, the full number of chromosomes is restored. If sperm and egg cells were produced by mitosis, then each successive generation would have twice the number of chromosomes as the preceding one.

The final step in the development of sperm is called spermiogenesis. In this process, the spermatids formed from spermatogenesis become mature spermatozoa, or sperm. The mature sperm cell has a head, midpiece, and tail. The head, also called the nuclear region, contains the 23 chromosomes surrounded by a nuclear membrane. The tip of the head is covered by an acrosome, which contains enzymes that help the sperm penetrate the female gamete. The midpiece, metabolic region, contains mitochondria that provide adenosine triphosphate (ATP). The tail, locomotor region, uses a typical flagellum for locomotion. The sperm are released into the lumen of the seminiferous tubule and leave the testes. They then enter the epididymis where they undergo their final maturation and become capable of fertilizing a female gamete.

Sperm production begins at puberty and continues throughout the life of a male. The entire process, beginning with a primary spermatocyte, takes about 74 days. After ejaculation, the sperm can live for about 48 hours in the female reproductive tract.

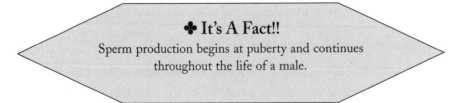

♣ It's A Fact!!
Sperm production begins at puberty and continues throughout the life of a male.

Duct System

Sperm cells pass through a series of ducts to reach the outside of the body. After they leave the testes, the sperm passes through the epididymis, ductus deferens, ejaculatory duct, and urethra.

Epididymis

Sperm leave the testes through a series of efferent ducts that enter the epididymis. Each epididymis is a long (about 6 meters) tube that is tightly coiled to form a comma-shaped organ located along the superior and posterior margins of the testes. When the sperm leave the testes, they are immature and incapable of fertilizing ova. They complete their maturation process and become fertile as they move through the epididymis. Mature sperm are stored in the lower portion, or tail, of the epididymis.

Ductus Deferens

The ductus deferens, also called vas deferens, is a fibromuscular tube that is continuous (or contiguous) with the epididymis. It begins at the bottom (tail) of the epididymis then turns sharply upward along the posterior margin of the testes. The ductus deferens enters the abdominopelvic cavity through the inguinal canal and passes along the lateral pelvic wall. It crosses over the ureter and posterior portion of the urinary bladder, and then descends along the posterior wall of the bladder toward the prostate gland. Just before it reaches the prostate gland, each ductus deferens enlarges to form an ampulla. Sperm are stored in the proximal portion of the ductus deferens, near the epididymis, and peristaltic movements propel the sperm through the tube.

The proximal portion of the ductus deferens is a component of the spermatic cord, which contains vascular and neural structures that supply the testes. The spermatic cord contains the ductus deferens, testicular artery and veins, lymph vessels, testicular nerve, cremaster muscle that elevates the testes for warmth and at times of sexual stimulation, and a connective tissue covering.

Ejaculatory Duct

Each ductus deferens, at the ampulla, joins the duct from the adjacent seminal vesicle (one of the accessory glands) to form a short ejaculatory duct.

Each ejaculatory duct passes through the prostate gland and empties into the urethra.

Urethra

The male urethra is divided into three regions. The prostatic urethra is the proximal portion that passes through the prostate gland. It receives the ejaculatory duct, which contains sperm and secretions from the seminal vesicles, and numerous ducts from the prostate glands. The next portion, the membranous urethra, is a short region that passes through the pelvic floor. The longest portion is the penile urethra (also called spongy urethra or cavernous ure-thra), which extends the length of the penis and opens to the outside at the external urethral orifice. The ducts from the bulbourethral glands open into the penile urethra.

♣ **It's A Fact!!**

The urethra extends from the urinary bladder to the external urethral orifice at the tip of the penis. It is a passageway for sperm and fluids from the reproductive system and urine from the urinary system. While reproductive fluids are passing through the urethra, sphincters contract tightly to keep urine from entering the urethra.

Accessory Glands

The accessory glands of the male reproductive system are the seminal vesicles, prostate gland, and the bulbourethral glands. These glands secrete fluids that enter the urethra.

Seminal Vesicles

The paired seminal vesicles are saccular glands posterior to the urinary bladder. Each gland has a short duct that joins with the ductus deferens at the ampulla to form an ejaculatory duct, which then empties into the urethra. The fluid from the seminal vesicles is viscous and contains fructose, which provides an energy source for the sperm; prostaglandins, which contribute to the mobility and viability of the sperm; and proteins that cause slight coagulation reactions in the semen after ejaculation.

Prostate

The prostate gland is a firm, dense structure that is located just inferior to the urinary bladder. It is about the size of a walnut and encircles the urethra as it leaves the urinary bladder. Numerous short ducts from the substance of the prostate gland empty into the prostatic urethra. The secretions of the prostate are thin, milky colored, and alkaline. They function to enhance the motility of the sperm.

Bulbourethral Glands

The paired bulbourethral (Cowper) glands are small, about the size of a pea, and located near the base of the penis. A short duct from each gland enters the proximal end of the penile urethra. In response to sexual stimulation, the bulbourethral glands secrete an alkaline mucus-like fluid. This fluid neutralizes the acidity of the urine residue in the urethra, helps to neutralize the acidity of the vagina, and provides some lubrication for the tip of the penis during intercourse.

Seminal Fluid

Seminal fluid, or semen, is a slightly alkaline mixture of sperm cells and secretions from the accessory glands. Secretions from the seminal vesicles make up about 60 percent of the volume of the semen, with most of the remainder coming from the prostate gland. The sperm and secretions from the bulbourethral gland contribute only a small volume.

The volume of semen in a single ejaculation may vary from 1.5 to 6.0 ml. There are usually between 50 to 150 million sperm per milliliter of semen. Sperm counts below 10 to 20 million per milliliter usually present fertility problems.

♣ It's A Fact!!

Although only one sperm actually penetrates and fertilizes the ovum, it takes several million sperm in an ejaculation to ensure that fertilization will take place.

Penis

The penis, the male copulatory organ, is a cylindrical pendant organ located anterior to the scrotum and functions to transfer sperm to the vagina. The penis consists of three columns of erectile tissue that are wrapped in connective tissue and covered with skin. The two dorsal columns are the corpora cavernosa. The single, midline ventral column surrounds the urethra and is called the corpus spongiosum.

The penis has a root, body (shaft), and glans penis. The root of the penis attaches it to the pubic arch, and the body is the visible, pendant portion. The corpus spongiosum expands at the distal end to form the glans penis. The urethra, which extends throughout the length of the corpus spongiosum, opens through the external urethral orifice at the tip of the glans penis. A loose fold of skin, called the prepuce, or foreskin, covers the glans penis.

Male Sexual Response

The male sexual response includes erection and orgasm accompanied by ejaculation of semen. Orgasm is followed by a variable time period during which it is not possible to achieve another erection.

Three hormones are the principle regulators of the male reproductive system. Follicle-stimulating hormone (FSH) stimulates spermatogenesis; luteinizing hormone (LH) stimulates the production of testosterone; and testosterone stimulates the development of male secondary sex characteristics and spermatogenesis.

Chapter 38

Circumcision

Definition

Circumcision is the surgical removal of the foreskin of the penis. It is often performed in healthy boys for cultural or religious reasons. In the U.S., a newborn boy is usually circumcised before he leaves the hospital. Jewish boys, however, are circumcised when they are eight days old.

Description

A numbing medication (local anesthesia) is usually applied before a circumcision to reduce pain. It might be injected at the base of the penis, in the shaft, or applied as a cream.

There are a variety of ways to perform a circumcision. Most commonly, the foreskin is pushed from the head of the penis and clamped with a metal or plastic ring-like device.

If the ring is metal, the foreskin is cut off and the metal device is removed. The wound heals in five to seven days.

If the ring is plastic, a piece of suture is tied tightly around the foreskin. This pushes the tissue into a groove in the plastic over the head of the penis. Within five to seven days, the plastic covering the penis falls free, leaving a completely healed circumcision.

The baby may be given a sweetened pacifier or lollipop during the procedure. Tylenol (acetaminophen) may be given afterward.

In older and adolescent boys, circumcision is usually done under general anesthesia while the child is completely asleep. The foreskin is removed and stitched onto the remaining skin of the penis. Stitches that dissolve (absorbable sutures) are used and will be absorbed within seven to ten days. The wound may take up to three weeks to heal.

Indications

In some faiths, including Judaism and Islam, circumcisions are performed on all baby boys as a religious rite. In other parts of the world, including Europe, Asia, and South and Central America, circumcision is rare in the general population.

> ♣ **It's A Fact!!**
> Rather than routinely recommending circumcision for healthy boys, many physicians allow the parents to make the decision after presenting them with the pros and cons.

The merits of circumcision are currently under debate, and opinions about the need for circumcision in healthy boys vary among physicians. Some place great value on the benefits of an intact foreskin, including a more natural sexual response during adulthood.

There is no compelling medical rationale for the procedure in healthy boys, although some boys have a medical condition requiring circumcision. However, some studies suggest that uncircumcised male infants have an increased risk of urinary tract infections. Other studies show correlations between being uncircumcised and an increased risk of developing penile cancer, certain sexually transmitted diseases including human immunodeficiency virus (HIV), infections of the penis, and phimosis (tightness of the foreskin that prevents it from retracting). The overall increased risk for these conditions is thought to be relatively small.

Proper hygiene of the penis and safe sexual practices can help prevent phimosis, penile cancer, acquired immune deficiency syndrome (AIDS), and other sexually transmitted diseases. Proper hygiene is always important but is thought to be especially important for uncircumcised males.

In 1999, the American Academy of Pediatrics revised their policy statement on circumcision, and this policy is supported by the American Medical Association. A summary of the policy is below:

"Existing scientific evidence demonstrates potential medical benefits of newborn male circumcision; however, these data are not sufficient to recommend routine neonatal circumcision. In circumstances in which there are potential benefits and risks, yet the procedure is not essential to the child's current well-being, parents should determine what is in the best interest of the child. To make an informed choice, parents of all male infants should be given accurate and unbiased information and be provided the opportunity to discuss this decision. If a decision for circumcision is made, procedural analgesia should be provided."

Risks

- Bleeding

- Infection

- Localized redness

- Injury to the penis

Expectations After Surgery

For both newborns and older children, circumcision is considered a very safe procedure.

Convalescence

Healing time for newborns after circumcision usually is about one week. Petroleum jelly (Vaseline) should be applied after changing the diaper to protect the healing incision. Some initial swelling and yellow crust formation around the incision is normal.

For older children and adolescents, healing may take up to three weeks. In most cases, the child will be discharged from the hospital on the day of the surgery. Home care for older children should include the following:

- Avoiding vigorous exercise during the healing.

- If the wound bleeds during the first 24 hours after surgery, pressure should be applied with a clean cloth for ten minutes.

- In older children, use ice packs (20 minutes on, 20 minutes off) for the first 24 hours after surgery to reduce swelling and pain. Bathing or showering is usually allowed. The incision may be gently washed with mild, unscented soap.

- Change the dressing at least once a day and apply an antibiotic ointment. If the dressing gets wet, change it promptly.

- Use prescribed pain medicine as directed. Pain medication should not be needed longer than four to seven days. In infants, use only acetaminophen, if needed.

Chapter 39

Is My Penis Normal?

Just about every guy wonders how he measures up in the "down there" department at one time or another. Here's the lowdown for any guy who's ever worried about whether his penis is a normal size.

Guys normally develop at different times. Some may start developing as early as 9. Others may not start developing until 15 or even later. The age at which a guy starts to grow varies from person to person. It all depends on when he enters puberty and his hormones start doing their thing.

Growth in penis size is just one part of puberty, which also includes such changes as pubic hair development, testicular growth, muscle development, and a growth spurt. Late starters almost always catch up fine— they just reach full maturity a little later.

Penises come in different sizes, shapes, and colors. These traits are hereditary, like eye color or foot size, and there's nothing you can do to change them. Despite what you may hear or read, no special exercises, supplements, or diets will speed up the development process or change a guy's size. Also, like his feet, a guy's penis may appear smaller to him just because the perspective is different when he's looking down. And there's a lot less difference

About This Chapter: This information was provided by TeensHealth, one of the largest resources online for medically reviewed health information written for parents, kids, and teens. For more articles like this one, visit www.TeensHealth.org, or www.KidsHealth.org. © 2005 The Nemours Foundation.

in penis size between guys when they get an erection (a "boner" or "hard on") than when their penises are relaxed.

In addition to size, guys also wonder about other aspects of how their penises look, such as whether the skin covering the penis is normal or if it's OK for a guy's penis to hang to the left or right (it is!). If you're concerned about how your penis looks, ask your doctor. Guys who are reaching puberty should have regular testicular exams, so that's a good time to ask your doctor any questions.

Taking a ride on the hormonal roller coaster means lots of changes—and a lot of common worries—for both guys and girls. Just as guys may wonder about how their penises develop, lots of girls ask the same thing about their breasts.

If you're wondering about your development, don't try to compare yourself to your older brother or your best friend—they're probably at a different stage of development than you are anyway. The important thing to remember is that it's OK to not be a mirror image of the guy at the next urinal.

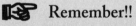 Remember!!

There's a fairly wide range of normal penis sizes—just as there is for every other body part. And just like other parts of the body, how a penis appears at different stages of a guy's life varies quite a bit. You wouldn't expect someone who is 11 years old to look the same as someone who's 19.

Chapter 40

Wet Dreams: A Guide To Nocturnal Emissions

The alarm clock sounds—time to wake up. You slowly open your eyes and try to figure out which pair of jeans you'll want to wear at school today. But wait, what's that? The bed sheets feel wet and sticky. The reality sets in.

For many of us, this scenario is all too real. Although most guys (and some girls) will at some point experience having a wet dream, many find the messy aftermath embarrassing. But having a wet dream is nothing to be ashamed of—in fact, it's totally natural and normal.

What's A Wet Dream?

A wet dream is an erotic dream that is so intense that a guy ejaculates (cums) in his sleep. Nocturnal emission is one of the ways the body gets rid of semen build up, so it usually doesn't happen during periods of masturbation or sex play. Very often guys don't remember the dream. If they don't know what's going on, they may think they've "wet the bed."

About This Chapter: Information in this chapter is from "Pleasant Dreams! A Guide to Nocturnal Emissions," reprinted with permission from Planned Parenthood® Federation of America, Inc. © 2007 PPFA. All rights reserved. For additional information, visit www.plannedparenthood.org.

Although wet dreams are most common among teenage guys, many men also have nocturnal emissions as adults. Some guys never have wet dreams, but most do. Dreams or no dreams—both are normal.

And ladies needn't feel left out—women and girls have wet dreams, too. Their vaginas become lubricated as they become sexually aroused in their dreams. But there is less evidence of wet dreams in women than in men because less liquid is produced or spilled on the bed sheets. Wet dreams are also more common in men, because a man's penis gets more tactile stimulation (physical touch) during sleep than a woman's clitoris.

What's Goin' On?

So what happens from the time you rest your eyes to the time your sheets get sticky? Here's how it works:

- During sleep, from time to time, our bodies enter periods called REM, or rapid eye movement, which last from a few minutes to a half hour.

> **☞ Remember!!**
> Having wet dreams is natural, normal, and nothing to be embarrassed about. In fact, many people believe that nocturnal emissions actually help to relieve stress. And on top of all that, they feel pretty good.

- During these sleep periods, guys experience several erections, and girls experience vaginal lubrication.

- If a dream during REM sleep is very arousing, the sensation of an erect penis pressed against a mattress can lead to erotic dreaming and ejaculation in guys. Girls can also have erotic dreams and get aroused to the point where they produce some liquid from their vaginas.

When It Gets Played Out

Having to change the sheets on a frequent basis can get annoying, and some guys may want to try to prevent wet dreams. In general, guys have nocturnal emissions less often if they are ejaculating while they are awake, either from masturbation or sex play with a partner. The same goes for girls who have wet dreams.

Of course, many girls and guys are perfectly content with their wet dreams. And that's fine too.

Chapter 41

Testicular Self-Exam

Performing a testicular self-exam can help detect cancer at an early, and very treatable, stage. Testicular cancer is the most common tumor in men between the ages of 29 and 35. If left untreated, testicular cancer may spread to the lymph nodes and lungs, where advanced cancer can be more difficult to treat successfully.

Self-examination is particularly important because cancer of the testes is asymptomatic. This means there are no symptoms such as fever or pain, which might clue you in to a potential health problem.

But here are a few warning signs such as the following:

- One testicle may swell or feel abnormally heavy.
- A small, painless lump may develop on a testicle.
- A dull ache in the lower abdomen or in the groin.
- Pain or discomfort in a testicle or in the scrotum.
- A sudden collection of fluid in the scrotum.
- Blood in the urine.
- Breasts may enlarge and feel tender.

About This Chapter: Information in this chapter is from "Testicular Self-Exam," © 2007 University of Ottawa Health Services. Reprinted with permission.

If you have lumps or other symptoms, it does not necessarily mean you have cancer. You need to go and see your doctor.

If detected and treated early, testicular cancer is one of the most curable cancers. (When caught early, 95% of cases are curable.) The treatment of testicular cancer usually does not end sexual activity. When discovered and treated early, it does not impair the individual's ability to have children. Waiting and hoping it will go away will not fix anything. If you're unsure, get checked out. It's worth your peace of mind.

You should examine yourself monthly using this procedure:

- Check yourself right after a warm bath or shower; the skin of the scrotum is then relaxed and soft.

- Stand in front of a mirror and check for any swelling on the scrotum skin. Become familiar with the normal size, shape, and weight of your testicles. One testicle may be slightly lower than the other, and one may be slightly larger. This is normal.

> ✔ **Quick Tip**
> Starting at around age 15, males should examine themselves every month.

- You should not feel any pain when doing the exam.

- Use both hands to examine each testicle. Gently roll the testicle between your fingers and thumb. Notice the epididymis, a rope-like structure on the top and back of each testicle, that stores and transports sperm. This structure is a normal part of the scrotum and not a tumor.

- Be on the alert for a tiny lump in the front, or along the sides of either testicle. A lump may feel like a kernel of uncooked popcorn or a small, hard pea.

- Report any swellings or lumps to a doctor right away.

Many men wait to see a doctor until cancer has spread and is more difficult to treat. This can be prevented by examining yourself.

Chapter 42

Testicular Cancer

What is testicular cancer?

Testicular cancer is a disease in which cells become malignant (cancerous) in one or both testicles.

The testicles (also called testes or gonads) are a pair of male sex glands. They produce and store sperm and are the main source of testosterone (male hormones) in men. These hormones control the development of the reproductive organs and other male physical characteristics. The testicles are located under the penis in a sac-like pouch called the scrotum.

Based on the characteristics of the cells in the tumor, testicular cancers are classified as seminomas or nonseminomas. Other types of cancer that arise in the testicles are rare and are not described here. Seminomas may be one of three types: classic, anaplastic, or spermatocytic. Types of nonseminomas include choriocarcinoma, embryonal carcinoma, teratoma, and yolk sac tumors. Testicular tumors may contain both seminoma and nonseminoma cells.

Testicular cancer accounts for only one percent of all cancers in men in the United States. About 8,000 men are diagnosed with testicular cancer, and about 390 men die of this disease each year.

About This Chapter: Information in this chapter is from "Testicular Cancer: Questions and Answers," the National Cancer Institute, U.S. National Institutes of Health, May 2005.

It is most common in white men, especially those of Scandinavian descent. The testicular cancer rate has more than doubled among white men in the past 40 years but has only recently begun to increase among black men. The reason for the racial differences in incidence is not known.

What are the risk factors for testicular cancer?

The exact causes of testicular cancer are not known. However, studies have shown that several factors increase a man's chance of developing this disease. They are as follows:

♣ **It's A Fact!!**
Testicular cancer occurs most often in men between the ages of 20 and 39 and is the most common form of cancer in men between the ages of 15 and 34.

- **Undescended Testicle (Cryptorchidism):** Normally, the testicles descend from inside the abdomen into the scrotum before birth. The risk of testicular cancer is increased in males with a testicle that does not move down into the scrotum. This risk does not change even after surgery to move the testicle into the scrotum. The increased risk applies to both testicles.

- **Congenital Abnormalities:** Men born with abnormalities of the testicles, penis, or kidneys, as well as those with inguinal hernia (hernia in the groin area, where the thigh meets the abdomen), may be at increased risk.

- **History Of Testicular Cancer:** Men who have had testicular cancer are at increased risk of developing cancer in the other testicle.

- **Family History Of Testicular Cancer:** The risk for testicular cancer is greater in men whose brother or father has had the disease.

How is testicular cancer detected? What are the symptoms of testicular cancer?

Doctors generally examine the testicles during routine physical exams. Between regular checkups, if a man notices anything unusual about his testicles, he should talk with his doctor. Men should see a doctor if they notice any of the following symptoms:

- A painless lump or swelling in a testicle

- Pain or discomfort in a testicle or in the scrotum

- Any enlargement of a testicle or change in the way it feels

- A feeling of heaviness in the scrotum

- A dull ache in the lower abdomen, back, or groin

- A sudden collection of fluid in the scrotum

These symptoms can be caused by cancer or by other conditions. It is important to see a doctor to determine the cause of any of these symptoms.

How is testicular cancer diagnosed?

✦ It's A Fact!!
Most testicular cancers are found by men themselves.

To help find the cause of symptoms, the doctor evaluates a man's general health. The doctor also performs a physical exam and may order laboratory and diagnostic tests. These tests include the following:

- **Blood tests** that measure the levels of tumor markers. Tumor markers are substances often found in higher-than-normal amounts when cancer is present. Tumor markers such as alpha-fetoprotein (AFP), beta-human chorionic gonadotropin (BHCG), and lactate dehydrogenase (LDH) may suggest the presence of a testicular tumor, even if it is too small to be detected by physical exams or imaging tests.

- *Ultrasound,* a test in which high-frequency sound waves are bounced off internal organs and tissues. Their echoes produce a picture called a sonogram. Ultrasound of the scrotum can show the presence and size of a mass in the testicle. It is also helpful in ruling out other conditions, such as swelling due to infection or a collection of fluid unrelated to cancer.

- *Biopsy* (microscopic examination of testicular tissue by a pathologist) to determine whether cancer is present. In nearly all cases of suspected cancer, the entire affected testicle is removed through an incision in the groin. This procedure is called radical inguinal orchiectomy. In rare cases (for example, when a man has only one testicle), the surgeon performs an inguinal biopsy, removing a sample of tissue from the testicle through an incision in the groin and proceeding with orchiectomy only if the pathologist finds cancer cells. (The surgeon does not cut through the scrotum to remove tissue. If the problem is cancer, this procedure could cause the disease to spread.)

If testicular cancer is found, more tests are needed to find out if the cancer has spread from the testicle to other parts of the body. Determining the stage (extent) of the disease helps the doctor to plan appropriate treatment.

How is testicular cancer treated? What are the side effects of treatment?

Most men with testicular cancer can be cured with surgery, radiation therapy, and/or chemotherapy. The side effects depend on the type of treatment and may be different for each person.

> ### ♣ It's A Fact!!
> Although the incidence of testicular cancer has risen in recent years, more than 95 percent of cases can be cured. Treatment is more likely to be successful when testicular cancer is found early. In addition, treatment can often be less aggressive and may cause fewer side effects.

Seminomas and nonseminomas grow and spread differently and are treated differently. Nonseminomas tend to grow and spread more quickly; seminomas are more sensitive to radiation. If the tumor contains both seminoma and nonseminoma cells, it is treated as a nonseminoma. Treatment also depends on the stage of the cancer, the patient's age and general health, and other factors. Treatment is often provided by a team of specialists, which may include a surgeon, a medical oncologist, and a radiation oncologist.

There are three types of standard treatment.

Surgery: Surgery to remove the testicle through an incision in the groin is called a radical inguinal orchiectomy. Men may be concerned that losing a testicle will affect their ability to have sexual intercourse or make them sterile (unable to produce children). However, a man with one healthy testicle can still have a normal erection and produce sperm. Therefore, an operation to remove one testicle does not make a man impotent (unable to have an erection) and seldom interferes with fertility (the ability to produce children). For cosmetic purposes, men can have a prosthesis (an artificial testicle) placed in the scrotum at the time of their orchiectomy or at any time afterward.

Some of the lymph nodes located deep in the abdomen may also be removed (lymph node dissection). This type of surgery does not usually change a man's ability to have an erection or an orgasm, but it can cause problems with fertility if it interferes with ejaculation. Patients may wish to talk with their doctor about the possibility of removing the lymph nodes using a special nerve-sparing surgical technique that may preserve the ability to ejaculate normally.

Radiation Therapy: Radiation therapy (also called radiotherapy) uses high-energy rays to kill cancer cells and shrink tumors. It is a local therapy, meaning that it affects cancer cells only in the treated areas. External radiation (from a machine outside the body), aimed at the lymph nodes in the abdomen, is used to treat seminomas. It is usually given after surgery. Because nonseminomas are less sensitive to radiation, men with this type of cancer usually do not undergo radiation therapy.

Radiation therapy affects normal as well as cancerous cells. The side effects of radiation therapy depend mainly on the treatment dose. Common side effects include fatigue, skin changes at the site where the treatment is given, loss of appetite, nausea, and diarrhea. Radiation therapy interferes with sperm production, but many patients regain their fertility over a period of one to two years.

Chemotherapy: Chemotherapy is the use of anticancer drugs to kill cancer cells. When chemotherapy is given to testicular cancer patients, it is usually given as adjuvant therapy (after surgery) to destroy cancerous cells that may remain in the body. Chemotherapy may also be the initial treatment if the cancer is advanced; that is, if it has spread outside the testicle at the time of the diagnosis. Most anticancer drugs are given by injection into a vein.

Chemotherapy is a systemic therapy, meaning drugs travel through the bloodstream and affect normal as well as cancerous cells throughout the body. The side effects depend largely on the specific drugs and the doses. Common side effects include nausea, hair loss, fatigue, diarrhea, vomiting, fever, chills, coughing/shortness of breath, mouth sores, or skin rash. Other side effects include dizziness, numbness, loss of reflexes, or difficulty hearing. Some anticancer drugs also interfere with sperm production. Although the reduction in sperm count is permanent for some patients, many others recover their fertility.

Some men with advanced or recurrent testicular cancer may undergo treatment with very high doses of chemotherapy. These high doses of chemotherapy kill cancer cells, but they also destroy the bone marrow, which makes and stores blood cells. Such treatment can be given only if patients undergo a bone marrow transplant. In a transplant, bone marrow stem cells are removed from the patient before chemotherapy is administered. These cells are frozen temporarily and then thawed and returned to the patient through a needle (like a blood transfusion) after the high-dose chemotherapy has been administered.

Men with testicular cancer should discuss their concerns about sexual function and fertility with their doctor. It is important to know that men with testicular cancer often have fertility problems even before their cancer is treated. If a man has pre-existing fertility problems, or if he is to have treatment that might lead to infertility, he may want to ask the doctor about sperm banking (freezing sperm before treatment for use in the future). This procedure allows some men to have children even if the treatment causes loss of fertility.

Is follow-up treatment necessary? What does it involve?

Regular follow-up exams are extremely important for men who have been treated for testicular cancer. Like all cancers, testicular cancer can recur (come back). Men who have had testicular cancer should see their doctor regularly and should report any unusual symptoms right away. Follow up varies for different types and stages of testicular cancer.

Chapter 43

Testicular Injuries

It hurts to even think about it. A baseball takes an unexpected bounce when you're crouched and waiting to field a grounder, an opponent misses a kick on the soccer field and his foot has only one place to go, or you're speeding along on your bike and you hit a big bump. All result in one really painful thing—a shot to the testicles, one of the most tender areas on a guy's body. Testicular injuries are relatively uncommon, but guys should be aware that they can happen. So how can you avoid injury?

Why Do Testicular Injuries Happen And What Can You Do?

If you're a guy who plays sports, likes to lift weights and exercise a lot, or leads an all-around active life, you've probably come to find out that the testicles are kind of vulnerable and can be injured in a variety of ways. Because they hang in a sac outside the body (the scrotum), the testicles are not protected by bones and muscles like other parts of your reproductive system and most of your other organs. Also, the location of the testicles makes them prime targets to be accidentally struck on the playing field or injured during strenuous exercise and activity.

About This Chapter: This information was provided by TeensHealth, one of the largest resources online for medically reviewed health information written for parents, kids, and teens. For more articles like this one, visit www.TeensHealth.org, or www.KidsHealth.org. © 2004 The Nemours Foundation.

The good news is that because the testicles are loosely attached to the body and are made of a spongy material, they're able to absorb most collisions without permanent damage. Testicles, although sensitive, can bounce back pretty quickly and minor injuries rarely have long-term effects. Also, sexual function or sperm production will most likely not be affected if you have a testicular injury.

You'll definitely feel pain if your testicles are struck or kicked, and you might also feel nauseous for a short time. If it's a minor testicular injury, the pain should gradually subside in less than an hour and any other symptoms should go away. In the meantime, you can do a few things to help yourself feel better such as take pain relievers, lie down, gently support the testicles with supportive underwear, and apply ice packs to the area. At any rate, it's a good idea to avoid strenuous activity for a while and take it easy for a few days.

However, if the pain doesn't subside or you experience extreme pain that lasts longer than an hour; if you have swelling or bruising of the scrotum or a puncture of the scrotum or testicle; if you continue to have nausea and vomiting; or if you develop a fever, get to a doctor immediately. These are symptoms of a much more serious injury that needs to be addressed as soon as possible.

Serious Testicular Injuries

Examples of serious testicular injury are testicular torsion and testicular rupture. In the case of testicular torsion, the testicle twists around, cutting off its blood supply. This can happen due to a serious trauma to the testicles, strenuous activity, or even for no apparent reason.

Testicular torsion isn't common, but when it does happen, it most often occurs in guys ages 12 to 18. If it occurs, it is crucial to see a doctor as soon as possible—within six hours of the time the pain starts. Unfortunately, after six hours, there is a much greater possibility that complications could result, including reduced sperm production or the loss of the testicle. The problem may be fixed by a doctor manually untwisting the testicle. If that doesn't work, surgery will be necessary.

Testicular rupture can also happen, but it is a rare type of testicular trauma. This can happen when the testicle receives a forceful direct blow or when the testicle is crushed against the pubic bone (the bone that forms the front of the pelvis), causing blood to leak into the scrotum. Testicular rupture, like testicular torsion and other serious injuries to the testicles, causes extreme pain, swelling in the scrotum, nausea, and vomiting. To fix the problem, surgery is necessary to repair the ruptured testicle.

Seeing A Doctor

If you have to see a doctor, he or she will first need to know how long you have been experiencing pain and how severe your discomfort is. To rule out a hernia or other problem as the cause of the pain, the doctor will examine your abdomen and groin. In addition, the doctor will look at your scrotum for swelling, color, and damage to the skin and examine the testicle itself. Because infections of the reproductive system or urinary tract can sometimes cause similar pain, your doctor may do a urine test to rule out a urinary tract infection or infection of the reproductive organs.

Preventing Testicular Injuries

It's a good idea to take precautions to avoid testicular injuries, especially if you play sports, exercise a lot, or just live an all-around active life. Here are some tips to keep your testicles safe and sound:

- **Protect your testicles.** Always wear an athletic cup or athletic supporter when playing sports or participating in strenuous activity. Athletic cups are usually made of hard plastic, are worn over the groin area, and provide a good degree of shielding and safety for the testicles. Cups are best used when participating in sports where your testicles might get hit or kicked, like football, hockey, soccer, or karate. An athletic supporter, or jock strap, is basically a cloth pouch that you wear to keep your testicles close to your body. Athletic supporters are best used when participating in strenuous exercise, cycling, or doing any heavy lifting.

- **Check your fit.** Make sure the athletic cup and/or athletic supporter is the right size. Safety equipment that's too small or too big won't protect you as effectively.

- **Keep your doctor informed.** If you play sports, you probably have regular physical exams by a doctor. If you experience testicular pain even occasionally, talk to your doctor about it.

- **Be aware of the risks of your sport or activity.** If you play a sport or participate in an activity with a high risk of injury, talk to your coach or doctor about any additional protective gear you should use.

☞ **Remember!!**

Participating in sports and living an active life are great ways to stay fit and relieve stress. But it's important to make sure your testicles are protected. When you're exercising or playing sports, make sure that using protective gear is part of your routine and you'll be able to play hard without fear of testicular injury.

Chapter 44

Guys And Enlarged Breasts: Gynecomastia

Ah, puberty. It can be a very interesting time in a guy's life, what with all the changes going on. In fact, it seems like every day something on your body grows bigger or hair begins sprouting somewhere. Each day brings a new change or two, and it can sometimes feel like it's hard to keep up.

It doesn't happen to every guy, but one of these changes can be the development of breast tissue. It's called gynecomastia (pronounced: guy-nuh-ko-mas-tee-uh), and it's completely normal—and almost always temporary. So how exactly does a guy happen to develop breast tissue?

What Is Gynecomastia?

Gynecomastia is a condition in which breast tissue forms in guys, usually due to normal hormonal changes during puberty. Hormones are chemicals produced by your body's glands. In a guy, hormones produced in the testicles are responsible for the physical changes that begin to take place during puberty—facial hair, muscle development, a deepening of the voice, and the lengthening of the penis, for example. Guys and girls produce both androgens (hormones that help develop and maintain male characteristics) and estrogen (a hormone that is responsible for most female characteristics).

About This Chapter: Text in this chapter is from "I'm a Guy... so How Come I'm Developing Breasts?" This information was provided by TeensHealth, one of the largest resources online for medically reviewed health information written for parents, kids, and teens. For more articles like this one, visit www.TeensHealth.org, or www.KidsHealth.org. © 2007 The Nemours Foundation.

Guys have mostly androgens in their systems, but they also have small amounts of estrogen. In girls, breast growth is caused by high levels of estrogen. Normally, when going through puberty, a guy's production of androgens increases significantly, whereas estrogen production remains low.

However, sometimes guys produce enough estrogen during puberty that some breast tissue develops. Breast tissue growth in guys can appear on one or both sides of the chest, and the breast area can feel tender. This doesn't mean you're turning into a girl or anything. It's just a minor change in your hormones as you begin to grow into adulthood.

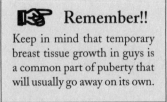

Remember!!

Keep in mind that temporary breast tissue growth in guys is a common part of puberty that will usually go away on its own.

It's estimated that about half of all males going through puberty experience some degree of gynecomastia in one or both breasts. Gynecomastia is almost always a temporary condition, and it's very unusual for the breasts to stay developed—they will eventually flatten out completely within a few months to a couple of years. It usually goes away on its own and no medical treatment or surgery is needed.

Even though it's just a temporary change for most teens, some guys with gynecomastia feel embarrassed or self-conscious about their appearance. Many guys find that wearing loose-fitting shirts helps make the condition less noticeable until the breast tissue shrinks over time. Surgical removal of the breast tissue is an option in some cases. If a guy finds his gynecomastia is bothering him, he can talk to a doctor about it.

Although the most common cause of gynecomastia is puberty, it can sometimes be caused by certain diseases or side effects of some medications. Using illegal drugs such as anabolic steroids, marijuana, or heroin can also disrupt hormonal balance and lead to gynecomastia.

There's also something called pseudogynecomastia (or false gynecomastia). This has nothing to do with puberty or hormones. It's just simply due to the fact that some guys have extra fat in the chest area, making it look like they have breasts. A doctor's exam can tell whether a guy has gynecomastia or pseudogynecomastia.

If you're concerned or have any questions about gynecomastia, talk to your doctor.

Chapter 45

Klinefelter Syndrome

What is Klinefelter syndrome?

Klinefelter syndrome, also known as the XXY condition, is a term used to describe males who have an extra X chromosome in most of their cells. Instead of having the usual XY chromosome pattern that most males have, these men have an XXY pattern.

Klinefelter syndrome is named after Dr. Henry Klinefelter, who first described a group of symptoms found in some men with the extra X chromosome. Even though all men with Klinefelter syndrome have the extra X chromosome, not every XXY male has all of those symptoms.

Because not every male with an XXY pattern has all the symptoms of Klinefelter syndrome, it is common to use the term XXY male to describe these men, or XXY condition to describe the symptoms.

What are the symptoms of the XXY condition?

Not all males with the condition have the same symptoms or to the same degree. Symptoms depend on how many XXY cells a man has, how much testosterone is in his body, and his age when the condition is diagnosed.

About This Chapter: National Institute of Child Health and Human Development, National Institutes of Health, May 2007.

The XXY condition can affect three main areas of development.

Physical Development: As babies, many XXY males have weak muscles and reduced strength. They may sit up, crawl, and walk later than other infants. After about age four, XXY males tend to be taller and may have less muscle control and coordination than other boys their age.

As XXY males enter puberty, they often do not make as much testosterone as other boys. This can lead to a taller, less muscular body, less facial and body hair, and broader hips than other boys. As teens, XXY males may have larger breasts, weaker bones, and a lower energy level than other boys.

> ♣ **It's A Fact!!**
> Scientists believe Klinefelter syndrome (the XXY condition) is one of the most common chromosome abnormalities in humans. About one of every 500 males has an extra X chromosome, but many don't have any symptoms.

By adulthood, XXY males look similar to males without the condition, although they are often taller. They are also more likely than other men to have certain health problems, such as autoimmune disorders, breast cancer, vein diseases, osteoporosis, and tooth decay.

XXY males can have normal sex lives, but they usually make little or no sperm. Between 95 percent and 99 percent of XXY males are infertile because their bodies do not make a lot of sperm.

Language Development: As boys, between 25 percent and 85 percent of XXY males have some kind of language problem, such as learning to talk late, trouble using language to express thoughts and needs, problems reading, and trouble processing what they hear.

As adults, XXY males may have a harder time doing work that involves reading and writing, but most hold jobs and have successful careers.

Social Development: As babies, XXY males tend to be quiet and undemanding. As they get older, they are usually quieter, less self-confident, less active, and more helpful and obedient than other boys.

As teens, XXY males tend to be quiet and shy. They may struggle in school and sports, meaning they may have more trouble "fitting in" with other kids.

However, as adults, XXY males live lives similar to men without the condition; they have friends, families, and normal social relationships.

What are the treatments for the XXY condition?

The XXY chromosome pattern cannot be changed, but there are a variety of ways to treat the symptoms of the XXY condition. They are as follows:

- **Educational Treatments:** As children, many XXY males qualify for special services to help them in school. Teachers can also help by using certain methods in the classroom, such as breaking bigger tasks into small steps.

- **Therapeutic Options:** A variety of therapists, such as physical, speech, occupational, behavioral, mental health, and family therapists, can often help reduce or eliminate some of the symptoms of the XXY condition, such as poor muscle tone, speech or language problems, or low self-confidence.

- **Medical Treatments:** Testosterone replacement therapy (TRT) can greatly help XXY males get their testosterone levels into normal range. Having a more normal testosterone level can help develop bigger muscles, deepen the voice, and grow facial and body hair. TRT often starts when a boy reaches puberty. Some XXY males can also benefit from fertility treatment to help them father children.

One of the most important factors for all types of treatment is starting it as early in life as possible.

Part Five

Pregnancy Prevention

Chapter 46

Teen Pregnancy Facts

Overview

- More than 800,000 teenagers become pregnant each year.

- Thirty-four percent of girls become pregnant at least once before age 20.

- Eleven percent of pregnant 15–17-year-olds have already been pregnant at least once before.

- Twenty percent of teens are sexually active before the age of 15, and 14% of these teens with early sexual debut will become pregnant during their teen years.

- Adolescent pregnancy is associated with higher rates of illness and death for both the mother and infant. Teenage girls are less emotionally and physically capable of having a healthy baby.

- Pregnant teens are at higher risk of having serious medical complications such as toxemia, hypertension, anemia, premature delivery, and placenta previa.

About This Chapter: Information in this chapter is from "Nonmarital Pregnancy," © Medical Institute for Sexual Health (www.medinstitute.org). Reprinted with permission. This undated information was reviewed for currency in 2007.

- The maternal death rate for mothers less than 15 years is greater than that of women in their 20s and is three times as high for unmarried women as for married women.

- Female teens are extremely fertile, and nearly 85% of teen pregnancies are unplanned.

- More than 90% of sexually active teens who do not use any form of contraception will become pregnant within one year of sexual debut, while 20% of teens less than 18 years who use condoms for contraception will become pregnant within one year of sexual activity.

- Nearly 50% of cohabiting female teens will become pregnant in the first year of contraceptive use.

What Happens To Teen Fathers?

In the timetable for the traditional transition from childhood to adolescence to adulthood, young people complete their high school education, may continue their education by attending college or completing specialized school or training, enter the labor force, marry, and become parents.

Teen fathers enter the labor market earlier, and initially earn more money, than do other males; but by the time teen fathers reach their mid-20s, they earn less.

> **♣ It's A Fact!!**
> For the teen, pregnancy is associated with serious health and emotional problems, poverty, low education, and single parenthood.

A study of teen fathers both before and after they become parents found they differed significantly from their peers—they were less likely to see themselves as being in control of their lives, both before and after they became parents.

What Happens To Teen Mothers?

At the individual level, nonmarital pregnancies to teens have a variety of consequences for teens and their children.

Pregnant adolescents are at increased risk for complications including low birth weight, infant mortality, preterm delivery, urinary tract infections, pyelonephritis, preeclampsia, and abortion. Unmarried teens (but not married teens) who become mothers are at increased risk for depressive symptoms later in life.

Nonmarital teen births often begin and end in poverty for the adolescent mother and her child/children. A majority (83%) of teen pregnancies, regardless of the outcome (birth, abortion, miscarriage), occur in economically disadvantaged areas. According to a 1998 report, nearly one-third of all teen mothers and one-half of unmarried teen mothers go on welfare within one year of giving birth. Almost a third (28%) of teen mothers are poor in their 20s and 30s, and 7% remain poor throughout the rest of their lives.

In general, teen mothers have much lower levels of educational attainment than other women, which severely limit their career options and sharply increase their likelihood of economic dependency. Only 70% of teen mothers complete high school or earn a GED [general education development], and far fewer—1.5%—earn a college degree by the age of 30.

The risk that a female will become a single parent is particularly high under 20 years of age. Ninety-seven percent of all births to girls under 15 are nonmarital, and 80% of births to 15- to 19-year-olds are nonmarital.

What Happens To Children Of Teen Parents?

For the child, there are also potential health problems, neglect, poverty, low education, incarceration, and drug use.

Children born to adolescent females are at increased risk for both prematurity and low birth weight. Low birth weight is associated with "infant death, blindness, deafness, respiratory problems, mental retardation, mental illness, cerebral palsy, dyslexia, and hyperactivity."

Children born to adolescent mothers are twice as likely to be the victim of neglect as those born to 20- or 21-year-old women.

The majority of teen mothers (80%) receive some form of public assistance, such as food stamps, Women, Infants, and Children (WIC) vouchers, or housing assistance. Half of all teenage mothers, and more than three-quarters of unmarried teen mothers, are on welfare within five years of giving birth.

Children of teenage mothers score lower on standard intelligence tests and achievement evaluations. Children of teen mothers are at increased risk of being placed in special education classes, probably due to factors associated with teenage pregnancies (that is, marital status, poverty). By three years of age, children of mothers born to adolescents show declines in mental functioning, delays in receptive language skills, and poor motor and social skills. Reasons may include lack of support form a social network and cognitive and emotional immaturity leading to an insecure mother-infant attachment.

Behavior problems are also common in children born to adolescents. Compared to children from two parent homes, the generation born to teen mothers is at increased risk for incarceration and drug use.

Chapter 47

Pregnancy Prevention Programs: Abstinence Versus Comprehensive Sex Education

Summary

The long-awaited experimentally designed evaluation of abstinence-only education programs, commissioned by Congress in 1997, indicates that young persons who participated in the U.S. Department of Health and Human Services' Title V Abstinence Education block grant program were no more likely than other young persons to abstain from sex. The evaluation conducted by Mathematica Policy, Inc. found that program participants had just as many sexual partners as non-participants, had sex at the same median age as non-participants, and were just as likely to use contraception as participants. For many analysts and researchers, the study confirms that a comprehensive sex education curriculum with an abstinence message and information about contraceptives and decision-making skills is a better approach to preventing teen pregnancy. Others maintain that the evaluation examined only four programs for elementary and middle school students and is thereby inconclusive. Separate experimentally designed evaluations of comprehensive sexual education programs found that some comprehensive

About This Chapter: Information in this chapter is excerpted from "Scientific Evaluations of Approaches to Prevent Teen Pregnancy," by Carmen Solomon-Fears, *CRS Report for Congress*, Order Code RS22656, May 1, 2007.

programs, including contraception information, decision-making skills, and peer pressure strategies, were successful in delaying sexual activity, improving contraceptive use, and/or preventing teen pregnancy.

Introduction

For many years, there have been divergent views with regard to sex and young persons. Many argue that sexual activity in and of itself is wrong if the persons are not married. Others agree that it is better for teenagers to abstain from sex, but are primarily concerned about the negative consequences of sexual activity, namely unintended pregnancy and sexually transmitted diseases (STDs). These two viewpoints are reflected in two teen pregnancy prevention approaches. The abstinence-only education approach centers on the abstinence-only message and exclusively funds programs

---

♣ It's A Fact!!
Abstinence-Only Education Inadequate, Says Study

Abstinence-only education has little to no impact on whether teens have sex or how many sexual partners they have, according to a new government study.

In 2005 and 2006, researchers surveyed 1,209 teens who had completed abstinence-only programs in rural and urban areas and 848 teens in the same communities who had not. The study found that teens in both groups reported practically identical sexual behavior.

Teens who took abstinence-only classes:

- were just as likely as teens in the other group to say they'd chosen not to be sexually active—about half remained abstinent in both groups

- had the same number of sexual partners as the teens that didn't take the classes— about a quarter said they'd had three or more partners and 27% had had one or two

- started having sex, on average, around the same age as those in the other group— 14.9 years old

- had unprotected sex just as often—21% in both groups said they sometimes or never used a condom

that adhere solely to bolstering that message. The Title V Abstinence Education block grant administered by the Department of Health and Human Services (HHS) supports this approach. The comprehensive sexual education approach provides funding (through many other federal programs) for both prevention programs (that often include an abstinence message) and programs that provide medical and social services to pregnant or parenting teens.

Abstinence-Only Education

A Title V Abstinence Education program (1) has, as its exclusive purpose, teaching the social, psychological, and health gains of abstaining from sexual activity; (2) teaching abstinence from sexual activity outside of marriage as the expected standard for all school-age children; (3) teaching that abstinence is the

The study, conducted by the nonpartisan research group Mathematica Policy Research, Inc., and funded by the federal government, focused on four programs that lasted from one to four years. On average, the kids were 11 to 12 years old when they entered the programs.

It should be noted that the abstinence education programs involved in the study represent just a few of the first programs established. Hundreds now are offered nationwide. None of the programs studied extended into the later high school years, when teens are more sexually active.

The American Academy of Pediatrics (AAP) recommends sex education programs that address abstinence and birth control. Research has shown that giving kids information about both options doesn't increase their sexual activity. For sexually active teens it promotes and increases the proper use of birth control methods.

Source: This information was provided by KidsHealth, one of the largest resources online for medically reviewed health information written for teens, kids, and parents. For more articles like this one, visit www.KidsHealth.org, or www.TeensHealth.org. © 2007 The Nemours Foundation.

Definitions

✎ What's It Mean?

Abstinence-Only Education teaches abstinence as the only morally correct option of sexual expression for teenagers. It usually censors information about contraception and condoms for the prevention of sexually transmitted diseases (STDs) and unintended pregnancy.

Abstinence-Only-Until-Marriage Education teaches abstinence as the only morally correct option of sexual expression for unmarried young people. Programs funded under the 1996 Welfare Reform Act must censor information about contraception and condoms for the prevention of STDs and unintended pregnancy.

Abstinence-Centered Education is another term normally used to mean abstinence-only education.

Comprehensive Sex Education teaches about abstinence as the best method for avoiding STDs and unintended pregnancy but also teaches about condoms and contraception to reduce the risk of unintended pregnancy and of infection with STDs, including HIV. It also teaches interpersonal and communication skills and helps young people explore their own values, goals, and options.

Abstinence-Based Education is another term normally used to mean comprehensive sexuality education.

Abstinence-Plus Education is another term normally used to mean comprehensive sexuality education.

Comparing Sex Education Programs

Comprehensive Sex Education

- teaches that sexuality is a natural, normal, healthy part of life

- teaches that abstinence from sexual intercourse is the most effective method of preventing unintended pregnancy and sexually transmitted diseases including HIV

- provides values-based education and offers students the opportunity to explore and define their individual values as well as the values of their families and communities

- includes a wide variety of sexuality related topics such as human development, relationships, interpersonal skills, sexual expression, sexual health, and society and culture

- includes accurate, factual information on abortion, masturbation, and sexual orientation

- provides positive messages about sexuality and sexual expression including the benefits of abstinence

- teaches that proper use of latex condoms, along with water-based lubricants, can greatly reduce, but not eliminate, the risk of unintended pregnancy and of infection with sexually transmitted diseases (STDs) including HIV

- teaches that consistent use of modern methods of contraception can greatly reduce a couple's risk for unintended pregnancy

- includes accurate medical information about STDs including HIV; teaches that individuals can avoid STDs

- teaches that religious values can play an important role in an individual's decisions about sexual expression; offers students the opportunity to explore their own and their family's religious values

- teaches that a woman faced with an unintended pregnancy has options: carrying the pregnancy to term and raising the baby, or carrying the pregnancy to term and placing the baby for adoption, or ending the pregnancy with an abortion

Abstinence-Only-Until-Marriage Education

- teaches that sexual expression outside of marriage will have harmful social, psychological, and physical consequences

- teaches that abstinence from sexual intercourse before marriage is the only acceptable behavior

- teaches only one set of values as morally correct for all students

- limits topics to abstinence-only-until-marriage and to the negative consequences of premarital sexual activity

- usually omits controversial topics such as abortion, masturbation, and sexual orientation

continued on next page

*Comparing Sex Education Programs: Abstinence-Only-Until-Marriage
Education, continued from previous page*

- often uses fear tactics to promote abstinence and to limit sexual expression

- discusses condoms only in terms of failure rates; often exaggerates condom failure rates

- provides no information on forms of contraception other than failure rates of condoms

- often includes inaccurate medical information and exaggerated statistics regarding STDs including HIV; suggests that STDs are an inevitable result of premarital sexual behavior

- often promotes specific religious values

- teaches that carrying the pregnancy to term and placing the baby for adoption is the only morally correct option for pregnant teens

Source: "Sex Education Programs: Definitions and Point-by-Point Comparison,"
© 2001 Advocates for Youth. All rights reserved. Reprinted with permission.

only certain way to avoid out-of-wedlock pregnancy, STDs, and associated health problems; (4) teaching that a mutually faithful monogamous relationship within marriage is the expected standard of human sexual activity; (5) teaching that sexual activity outside of marriage is likely to have harmful psychological and physical effects; (6) teaching that bearing children out-of-wedlock is likely to have harmful consequences for the child, the child's parents, and society; (7) teaching young people how to reject sexual advances and how alcohol and drug use increases vulnerability to sexual advances; and (8) teaching the importance of attaining self-sufficiency before engaging in sex.

Comprehensive Sexual Education

Advocates of a more comprehensive approach to sex education argue that today's youth need information and decision-making skills to make realistic, practical choices about whether to engage in sexual activities. They contend that such an approach allows young people to make informed decisions regarding abstinence, gives them the information they need to resist peer pressure and to set relationship limits, and also provides them with information on prevention of STDs and the use of contraceptives.

Many analysts and researchers agree that effective pregnancy prevention programs have many of the following characteristics:

- Convince teens that not having sex or that using contraception consistently and carefully is the right thing to do

- Last a sufficient length of time

- Are operated by leaders who believe in their programs and who are adequately trained

- Actively engage participants and personalize the program information

- Address peer pressure

- Teach communication skills

- Reflect the age, sexual experience, and culture of young persons in the programs

Although there have been numerous evaluations of teen pregnancy prevention programs, there are many reasons why programs are not considered successful. In some cases, the evaluation studies are limited by methodological problems or constraints because the approach taken is so multilayered that researchers have had difficulty disentangling the effects of multiple components of a program. In other cases, the approach may have worked for boys but not for girls, or vice versa. In some cases the programs are very small, and thereby it is harder to obtain significant results. In other cases, different personnel may affect the outcomes of similar programs.

An Abstinence-Only Intervention Versus An Abstinence Message

There is a significant difference between abstinence as a message and abstinence-only interventions. While the Bush Administration continues to support an abstinence-only program intervention (with some modifications), others argue that an abstinence message integrated into a comprehensive sex education program that includes information on the use of contraceptives and that enhances decision-making skills is a more effective method to prevent teen pregnancy. A recent nationally representative survey found that 90% of adults and teens agree that young people should get a strong message that they should not have sex until they are at least out of high school, and that a majority of adults (73%) and teens (56%) want teens to get more information about both abstinence and contraception. The American public—both adults and teens—supports encouraging teens to delay sexual activity and providing young people with information about contraception.

Chapter 48

Rhythm Method

What Is It?

The rhythm method is a way to prevent pregnancy by not having sex around the time of ovulation (the release of an egg during a girl's monthly cycle). Couples who do want to have a baby can also use this method to have sex during the time that they are most likely to conceive. It is sometimes called natural family planning, periodic abstinence, or fertility awareness.

How Does It Work?

If a couple doesn't have sex around the time of ovulation, the girl can't get pregnant. The trick is knowing when ovulation happens. Couples use a calendar, a thermometer to measure body temperature, a kit that tests the thickness of cervical mucus, or a kit that tests for ovulation. The ovulation kits are more useful for couples who are trying to get pregnant. The fertile period around ovulation lasts six to nine days, and during this time the couple should not have unprotected sex.

About This Chapter: Text in this chapter is from "Birth Control: Rhythm Method." This information was provided by TeensHealth, one of the largest resources online for medically reviewed health information written for parents, kids, and teens. For more articles like this one, visit www.TeensHealth.org, or www.KidsHealth.org. © 2007 The Nemours Foundation.

How Well Does It Work?

Over the course of one year, as many as 25 out of 100 typical couples who rely on the rhythm method to prevent pregnancy will have an accidental pregnancy. Of course, this is an average figure, and the chance of getting pregnant depends on whether a couple uses one or more of the rhythm method tools correctly and consistently and that they do not have unprotected sex during the fertile period.

In general, how well each type of birth control method works depends on a lot of things. These include whether a person has any health conditions, is taking any medications that might interfere with its use, whether the method chosen is convenient—and whether it is used correctly all the time. In the case of the rhythm method, it also depends on how consistent a woman's ovulatory cycle is and how accurately a couple keeps track of when she could be ovulating.

Protection Against STDs

The rhythm method does not protect against sexually transmitted diseases (STDs). Couples having sex must always use condoms along with their chosen method of birth control to protect against STDs.

Abstinence (not having sex) is the only method that always prevents pregnancy and STDs.

Who Uses It?

The rhythm method is not a reliable way to prevent pregnancy for most teens. It is often very difficult to tell when a girl is fertile, and she can conceive for up to six days before she ovulates to one or two days after. Because teens often have irregular menstrual cycles, it makes predicting ovulation much more difficult. The rhythm method requires a commitment to monitoring body changes, keeping daily records, and above all not having sex during the fertile period. Couples often need to practice for months to get this method right.

How Do You Get It?

For couples interested in this method, it is best to talk to a doctor or counselor who is trained in fertility awareness. He or she can then teach the couple the skills they need to know to practice the rhythm method accurately.

How Much Does It Cost?

The tools needed for the rhythm method—such as ovulation detection kits and thermometers, for example—are available in drugstores but can be expensive. Again, it's best to talk to a doctor for advice on using this method.

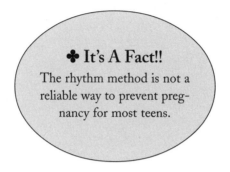

♣ It's A Fact!!
The rhythm method is not a reliable way to prevent pregnancy for most teens.

Chapter 49

Male Condom

What is a male condom?

The male condom is a sheath that is rolled over the penis to prevent semen from entering the vagina. Condoms are a barrier method of birth control made of latex, polyurethane, or lambskin, to be disposed of after each use.

How does a male condom work?

Most male condoms have a small reservoir at the tip of the condom used to catch the sperm during ejaculation. The male condom reduces the likelihood that the vagina and cervix will come in direct contact with the penis or with secretions from the penis. Some condoms come with a spermicidal agent designed to kill the sperm.

According to the Mayo Clinic, 2 out of every 100 condoms break. Lubrications may be used to help prevent condoms from tearing, but not all lubricants are safe to use with latex condoms.

How effective is a male condom?

The typical use of male condoms, which is the average way most people use them, has a failure rate of 14–15%. This means that 14–15 people out of every 100 will become pregnant during the first year of use. Spermicidal agents increase the effectiveness to over 95% when used correctly and consistently. You should take a pregnancy test if you are experiencing any pregnancy symptoms.

What are the side effects or health risks of male condoms?

Male condoms do not have any side effects except to individuals who are allergic to latex.

Condom Dos And Don'ts   ✔ Quick Tip

- Use lubricated latex condoms. Always use latex, because lambskin condoms do not block human immunodeficiency virus (HIV) and sexually transmitted diseases (STDs), and polyurethane condoms break more often than latex. Shop around and find your favorite brand. Try different sizes and shapes (yes, they come in different sizes and shapes). There are a lot of choices. One will work for you.

- Store condoms loosely in a cool, dry place (not your wallet). Make sure your condoms are fresh. Check the expiration date. Throw away condoms that have expired, been very hot, or been washed in the washer. If you think the condom might not be good, get a new one. You and your partner are worth it.

- Open the package carefully, so that you do not rip the condom. Be careful if you use your teeth. Make sure that the condom package has not been punctured (there should be a pocket of air). Check the condom for damaged packaging and signs of aging such as brittleness, stickiness, and discoloration.

- Put on the condom after the penis is erect and before it touches any part of a partner's body. If a penis is uncircumcised (uncut), the foreskin must be pulled back before putting on the condom.

- Make sure the condom is right-side out. It is like a sock. There is a right side and a wrong side. Before you put it on the penis, unroll the condom about half an inch to see which direction it is unrolling. Then put it on the head of the penis and hold the tip of the condom between

Is a male condom reversible?

Yes. It is possible to get pregnant immediately if condoms are no longer used.

How much does a male condom cost?

The cost of male condoms depends on the style (ribbed, lubricated) and the type (latex, lambskin, polyurethane). Most condoms are purchased in packages from 3 to 12. The cost per condom ranges from as little as 20¢ to $2.50 each. Some health facilities may distribute condoms free.

---

your fingers as you roll it all the way down the shaft of the penis from head to base. This keeps out air bubbles that can cause the condom to break. It also leaves a space for semen to collect after ejaculation.

- If you use a lubricant (lube), it should be a water-soluble lubricant (for example, ID Glide, K-Y Jelly, Slippery Stuff, Foreplay, Wet, Astroglide) in order to prevent breakdown of the condom. Products such as petroleum jelly, massage oils, butter, Crisco, Vaseline, and hand creams are not considered water-soluble lubricants and should not be used.

- Put lubricant on after you put on the condom, not before. It could slip off. Add more lube often. Dry condoms break more easily.

- Withdraw the penis immediately after ejaculation, while the penis is still erect. Grasp the rim of the condom between your fingers and slowly withdraw the penis (with the condom still on) so that no semen is spilled.

- Throw out the used condom right away. Tie it off to prevent spillage or wrap it in bathroom tissue and put it in the garbage. Condoms can clog toilets. Use a condom only once. Never use the same condom for vaginal and anal intercourse. Never use a condom that has been used by someone else.

Source: Excerpted from "Tips for Using Condoms and Dental Dams," Tips and Tools, National HIV/AIDS Program, United States Department of Veterans Affairs, March 2007.

♣ It's A Fact!!

Benefits Of Condom Use At Sexual Debut Go Beyond Contraception

Several years after sexual debut, early condom users had lower sexually transmitted infection (STI) rates than did nonusers.

Several studies have shown that condom use at sexual debut is associated with continued condom use. To assess the relation between condom use at first vaginal coitus with rates of sexually transmitted infections (STIs), investigators analyzed data from more than 4,000 sexually active participants (52% women; average age of all participants at sexual debut, 15.2) in the National Longitudinal Study of Adolescent Health. Beginning in 1994, the investigators conducted three waves of in-home interviews; at the time of the third wave (when the average age of participants was 22.2), urine samples were collected and tested with ligase chain reaction (LCR) for *Neisseria gonorrhoeae* and *Chlamydia trachomatis* DNA.

In comparisons adjusted for factors such as socioeconomic status, education level, and risk-taking characteristics, condom users at initial coitus were 36% more likely to have used a condom at their most recent coitus (P less than 0.01) and half as likely to test positive for *C. trachomatis* or *N. gonorrhoeae* (P less than 0.05) compared with non-condom users. The number of sexual partners was similar in the two groups.

Comment: By making adjusted comparisons, the authors have addressed the possibility that initial condom users simply are not risk takers in general. Given that the adjustment had little effect and that the number of sexual partners was similar between the groups, that explanation is not likely. The authors conclude that initial condom use is an independent factor associated with healthy outcomes many years later. A unique strength of this study is the authors' use of LCR as a biomarker to validate self-reported sexual behavior. A reduction in STI rates of this magnitude is nothing short of amazing. Promoting abstinence should always be our first line—but these results show that all adolescents should also be educated about condom use and availability so that if they choose to become sexually active, they will have the means to use condoms at first coitus.

Source: Ann Davis, MD. "Benefits of Condom Use at Sexual Debut Go Beyond Contraception." *Journal Watch Women's Health*, Vol. 12, No. 9, p. 65, September 2007. Copyright © 2007 Massachusetts Medical Society. All rights reserved.

What about male condoms and sexually transmitted diseases (STDs)?

A condom is the only means of birth control that provides any reduction in the transmission of sexually transmitted diseases. However condoms are not "safe sex," but rather "safer sex." According to the workshop summary, "Scientific Evidence on Condom Effectiveness for Sexually Transmitted Disease (STD) Prevention," July 2001, The National Institute of Health and the National Institute of Allergy and Infectious Diseases report the following:

- Condoms provide no reduction in the transmission of the human papilloma virus (HPV) or *Trichomonas vaginalis*.

- Syphilis transmission is reduced 29% for typical use. It is reduced 50 to 71% when condoms are used correctly 100% of the time.

- Gonorrhea and chlamydia transmission is reduced by approximately 50% even when condoms are used 100% of the time.

- Genital herpes transmission is reduced by approximately 40%.

- Human immunodeficiency virus (HIV) transmission is reduced by approximately 85% when condoms are used correctly 100% of the time.

Condoms help prevent the transmission of STDs by reducing the likelihood of partner exposure through genital contact or fluid secretions. Condoms only reduce the likelihood of exposure; they do not prevent exposure.

What are the pros and cons for male condoms?

The pros of male condoms include the following:

- It is one of the few forms of birth control that provides any reduction in the transmission of sexually transmitted diseases.

- Condoms are inexpensive and easily obtained.

- There are no side effects unless you are allergic to latex.

- You do not need a prescription.

- Condoms are small, easy to carry, and disposable.

The cons of male condoms include the following:

- Some men complain condoms dull sensations.

- They may be considered an interruption during intimate foreplay.

- They require consistent and diligent use.

- Typical use has a failure rate of approximately 14%.

- It places more responsibility on the male partner.

Chapter 50

Female Condom

What is a female condom?

The female condom is a pouch made of polyurethane or latex that fits inside the vagina. It is a barrier method of birth control.

How does a female condom work?

The female condom has a flexible ring at the closed end of the pouch with a slightly larger ring at the open end. The smaller ring at the closed end keeps the female condom in place, whereas the larger ring rests outside the vagina. The female condom keeps the vagina and cervix from coming in contact with the skin of the penis or with secretions from the penis.

How effective is a female condom?

The typical use of female condoms, which is the average way most people use them, has a failure rate of 21%. This means that 21 people out of every 100 will become pregnant during the first year of use. You may increase effectiveness by adding a spermicidal foam, jelly, or cream in conjunction with the condom. You should take a pregnancy test if you are experiencing any pregnancy symptoms.

About This Chapter: Reprinted with permission from the American Pregnancy Association, http://www.americanpregnancy.org, © 2005. All rights reserved.

What are the side effects or health risks of female condoms?

Female condoms do not have any side effects except to individuals who are allergic to latex.

Is a female condom reversible?

Yes. The female condom does not have any effects on either the male or the female reproductive function. It is possible to get pregnant immediately if condoms are no longer used.

How much does a female condom cost?

The cost of female condoms is higher than male condoms and both types are only used once. The cost ranges from as little as $2.50 to $5.00 each.

What about female condoms and sexually transmitted diseases (STDs)?

A condom is the only means of birth control that provides a significant reduction in the transmission of sexually transmitted diseases.

Condoms help prevent the transmission of STDs by reducing the likelihood of partner exposure through genital contact or fluid secretions.

The female condom has not been studied near as much as the male condom counterpart, but it provides similar properties.

Information about male condoms: According to the workshop summary, "Scientific Evidence on Condom Effectiveness for Sexually Transmitted Disease (STD) Prevention," July 2001, The National Institute of Health and the National Institute of Allergy and Infectious Diseases report:

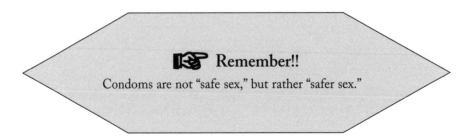

☞ Remember!!
Condoms are not "safe sex," but rather "safer sex."

- Condoms provide no reduction in the transmission of the human papilloma virus (HPV) and *Trichomonas vaginalis*.

- Syphilis transmission is reduced 29% for typical use. It is reduced 50 to 71% when condoms are used correctly 100% of the time.

- Gonorrhea and chlamydia transmission is reduced by approximately 50% even when condoms are used 100% of the time.

- Genital herpes transmission is reduced by approximately 40%.

- Human immunodeficiency virus (HIV) transmission is reduced by approximately 85% when condoms are used correctly 100% of the time.

What are the pros and cons for female condoms?

The pros of female condoms include:

- Along with male condoms, it is the only form of birth control that has a significant reduction in the transmission of sexually transmitted diseases.

- It keeps the control of contraceptive use in your hands.

- You do not need a prescription.

- Compared to the male condom, it is less likely to cause an allergic reaction, and it is less likely to break.

- Condoms are small, easy to carry, and disposable.

The cons of female condoms include:

- They are more expensive than male condoms (approximately five times).

- The outer ring may be considered cumbersome.

- Typical use has a higher failure rate of approximately 21%.

- It may be a distraction during intercourse because of crackling or popping noises.

Chapter 51

Diaphragm, Cervical Cap, And Cervical Shield

What They Are And How They Work

Diaphragms, caps, and shields are soft latex or silicone barriers that cover the cervix.

- The diaphragm is a shallow, dome shaped cup with a flexible rim. It fits securely in the vagina to cover the cervix.

- FemCap is a silicone cup shaped like a sailor's hat. It fits securely in the vagina to cover the cervix.

- Lea's Shield is a silicone cup with an air valve and a loop to aid in removal. It fits snugly over the cervix.

Each method must be used with spermicide cream or jelly.

Diaphragms, caps, and shields keep sperm from joining the egg.

- They block the opening to the uterus.

- The contraceptive cream or jelly stops sperm from moving.

About This Chapter: Information in this chapter is from "Diaphragms, Caps, and Shields," reprinted with permission from Planned Parenthood® Federation of America, Inc. © 2007 PPFA. All rights reserved. For additional information, visit www.plannedparenthood.org.

Effectiveness

Sixteen out of 100 women who use the diaphragm will become pregnant during the first year of typical use. * Six will become pregnant with perfect use. **

Fourteen out of 100 women who have never been pregnant or given birth vaginally and use FemCap will become pregnant during the first year of typical use. Of 100 women who have given birth vaginally and use FemCap, 29 will become pregnant during the first year of typical use. *** Effectiveness rates for perfect use are not available.

Fifteen out of 100 women who use the shield will become pregnant during the first year of typical use. Effectiveness rates for perfect use are not available.

Protection may be increased by:

• making sure the cervix is covered before each act of intercourse

• making sure spermicide is used as recommended

• using a latex condom

Diaphragms, caps, and shields offer no protection against sexually transmitted infection. Use a latex condom to reduce the risk of infection.

* Typical use refers to failure rates for women whose use is not consistent or always correct.

** Perfect use refers to failure rates for those whose use is consistent and always correct.

*** Effectiveness rates for FemCap are those for an earlier version of the device. Although no studies have been published yet, the manufacturers of FemCap report that the current device is likely to be more effective.

How To Get Them

You must see a health care provider. Your provider will examine you to make sure you do not have a condition that would rule out using a diaphragm, cap, or shield. Your provider will determine the correct size for diaphragms and caps and will provide information about use, insertion, and removal.

Diaphragms are available in many sizes and designs. A new size may be needed after any of the following:

- a full-term pregnancy

- abdominal or pelvic surgery

- a miscarriage or abortion after 14 weeks of pregnancy

- a 20 percent change in weight

FemCap is available in the following three sizes:

- small, for women who have never been pregnant

- medium, for women who have had an abortion or a cesarean delivery

- large, for women who have given birth vaginally

The shield only comes in one size.

Women should have regular pelvic examinations. It is a good idea to bring your diaphragm, cap, or shield to your examination.

> **✔ Quick Tip**
> **Practice Makes Perfect**
> The better a diaphragm, cap, or shield fits and is inserted, the better it will stay in place—and better protect against pregnancy. Your clinician will show you how to insert and remove your diaphragm, cap, or shield and will then watch you insert and remove it. Practice inserting and removing it at home, too.

Some Conditions That May Rule Out Use Of Diaphragms, Caps, And Shields

- allergy to latex, silicone, or spermicide

- childbirth in the last six weeks (ten weeks for FemCap)

- difficulty with insertion

- discomfort with touching one's genitals

- history of toxic shock syndrome

- recent cervical surgery

- recent abortion after the first trimester (after any recent abortion for FemCap)

- sagging uterus

- vaginal obstructions

A woman may not be able to use a diaphragm if she has:

- frequent urinary tract infections

- poor vaginal muscle tone

She may not be able to use FemCap if she has:

- breaks in the vaginal or cervical tissue

- cancer of the uterus, vagina, or vulva

- a reproductive tract infection

- poor vaginal muscle tone

She may not be able to use a shield if she has:

- breaks in the vaginal or cervical tissue

- frequent urinary tract infections

- a reproductive tract infection

Women should not use the diaphragm, cap, or shield during any kind of vaginal bleeding—including menstruation.

The diaphragm, cap, and shield are intended for each woman's use. Do not share them with friends.

Advantages And Disadvantages Of Diaphragms, Caps, And Shields

Advantages

- can be used during breastfeeding

- easily carried in pocket or purse

- generally cannot be felt by either partner

- immediately effective and reversible

- no effect on a woman's natural hormones

- no interruption of sex play—can be inserted hours ahead of time

Disadvantages

- cannot be used during menstruation

- may be difficult for some women to insert

- may be pushed out of place by some sexual positions, penis sizes, and thrusting techniques and angles

- must be in place every time a woman has vaginal intercourse

- diaphragms and caps may require refitting

Use of the spermicide nonoxynol-9 many times a day by people at risk for human immunodeficiency virus (HIV), or for anal sex, may irritate tissue and increase the risk of HIV and other sexually transmitted infections.

♣ **It's A Fact!!**
Special Advantages For Teens

Many teen women have vaginal intercourse only now and then. Many of them prefer to use a prescription barrier method on those occasions. That way they avoid the possible ongoing side effects of prescription methods with hormones.

Possible Side Effects

- Some women who use diaphragms and shields may develop frequent bladder infections. They should urinate before inserting the diaphragm or shield and after intercourse. A woman who gets frequent bladder infections should also have her clinician check the fit of her diaphragm.

- Women who are allergic to latex, silicone, or some brands of spermicide may not be able to use diaphragms, caps, or shields. Women who have a mild reaction to spermicide may try switching brands to clear up the problem.

- Some women or their partners may feel pain or discomfort when using FemCap or the shield.

Check with your clinician if you have:

- burning sensations while urinating

- discomfort when the diaphragm, cap, or shield is in place

- irregular spotting and bleeding

- irritation or itching in the genital area

- redness or swelling of the vulva or vagina

- unusual discharge from the vagina

How To Use The Diaphragm

- Wash hands with soap and water.

- Put about a tablespoon of spermicide in the cup. Spread some around the rim.

- Find a comfortable position—stand with one foot on a chair, sit on the edge of a chair, lie down, or squat.

- Separate the labia with one hand. Pinch the rim of the diaphragm to fold it in half with the other hand. Place index finger in the center of fold for a firmer grip. The spermicide must be inside the fold.

> ♣ It's A Fact!!
> **Toxic Shock Syndrome**
>
> Rare cases of toxic shock syndrome (TSS) have been reported with diaphragm use. The symptoms of TSS include:
>
> - a sunburn-type rash
> - diarrhea
> - dizziness, faintness, weakness
> - sore throat, aching muscles and joints
> - sudden high fever
> - vomiting
>
> If you have these symptoms, remove the diaphragm, cap, or shield and contact your clinician immediately.

- Push as far up and back in the vagina as possible. Tuck behind the pubic bone. Make sure the cervix is covered.

- It must stay in place six hours after the last act of intercourse.

- If intercourse is repeated or occurs more than six hours after insertion, leave the diaphragm in place and apply more spermicide.

- Do not leave the diaphragm in place for more than 24 hours.

- To remove, wash hands with soap and water. Hook a finger over the top of the rim to break the suction. Pull the diaphragm down and out.

- A special inserter can be used to help with placement and removal.

How To Use FemCap

- Wash hands with soap and water.

- Put one-quarter teaspoon of spermicide in the dome of FemCap, spread a thin layer on the brim, and put one-half teaspoon in the folded area between the brim and the dome.

- Find a comfortable position—stand with one foot on a chair, sit on the edge of a chair, lie down, or squat.

- Locate your cervix with index and middle fingers.

- Separate the labia with one hand and squeeze the rim together with the other.

- Slide FemCap into the vagina with the long brim entering first and the dome-side down. Push down towards the rectum and then up and onto the cervix. Make sure the cervix is completely covered. (Insertion is easier before sexual arousal).

- With each act of intercourse, check that FemCap is still covering the cervix. Apply more spermicide if you like.

- FemCap must stay in place six hours after the last intercourse.

- Do not leave FemCap in place for more than 48 hours.

- To remove, wash hands with soap and water. Squat down. Grip the removal strap and rotate FemCap. Push on the dome with your finger to break the suction. Hook your finger under the removal strap and pull the cap out.

How To Use The Shield

- Wash hands with soap and water.

- Coat the inside of the bowl around the hole, the front of the rim, and outer part of the valve with spermicide.

- Find a comfortable position—stand with one foot on a chair, sit on the edge of a chair, lie down, or squat.

- Separate the labia with one hand. Pinch the rim of the shield.

- Slide the shield into the vagina with the valve facing down and the thickest end inserted first.

- Push the shield up as far in the vagina as is possible and comfortable. Make sure that the loop is not sticking out of your vagina.

- The air between the cervix and shield will be vented out through the valve to create a proper fit. You can press on the valve a few times or walk a few steps after insertion to make sure that the air is removed.

- With each act of intercourse, check that the shield is still covering the cervix. Apply more spermicide if you like.

- The shield must stay in place eight hours after the last intercourse.

- Do not leave the shield in place for more than 48 hours.

- To remove, wash hands with soap and water. Squat down and relax the muscles in your vagina. Grasp the loop with your finger and rotate the shield slightly to break the suction. Or grasp the rim of the shield with your thumb and pointer finger. Pull the shield down and out of your vagina.

Care Of Diaphragms, Caps, And Shields

With proper care, the diaphragm and FemCap may last about two years, and the shield may last about six months.

- After removal, wash with mild soap and warm water.

- Allow to air dry.

- Do not use powders—they can cause infections. Never use oil-based lubricants— such as Vaseline or cold cream—with diaphragms. They damage latex.

Examine regularly for small holes or weak spots by holding the device up to the light. Gently stretch the latex of the diaphragm between your fingers. Fill the cup of the diaphragm or cap with water and look for leaks.

Diaphragms, caps, and shields can still be used if the rubber becomes discolored. But if the rubber puckers—especially near the rim—it has become too thin.

Where To Get Them And What They Cost

Visit Planned Parenthood, other family planning clinics, your health maintenance organization (HMO), or a private doctor for an exam and prescription. Diaphragms, caps, and shields may be purchased at a drugstore or clinic. An examination costs from $50 to $200. Diaphragms, caps, and shields average from $15 to $75. Spermicide jelly or cream costs from about $8 to $17 a kit.

Medicaid may cover these costs. Private health insurance coverage for birth control varies. Clinics may offer lower prices than private health care providers.

Chapter 52

Contraceptive Sponge

What is a contraceptive sponge?

The contraceptive sponge is a soft saucer-shaped device made from polyurethane foam. It is considered a barrier method of contraception.

How does a contraceptive sponge work?

The contraceptive sponge is designed to fit over the cervix and works in three ways to prevent pregnancy:

- It blocks the cervix, preventing semen from entering the uterus.
- The sponge contains spermicide, which kills sperm.
- The sponge absorbs the semen.

How effective is a contraceptive sponge?

When the contraceptive sponge is used correctly and consistently, it has about a 9% failure rate or almost one in ten. Typical use of the contraceptive sponge refers to the way that most people use it. The failure rate during typical use is approximately 16%. You should take a pregnancy test if you are experiencing any pregnancy symptoms.

About This Chapter: Reprinted with permission from the American Pregnancy Association, http://www.americanpregnancy.org, © 2003. All rights reserved.

What are the side effects or health risks of a contraceptive sponge?

The contraceptive sponge has been associated with some women experiencing toxic shock syndrome (TSS)—a rare but serious life-threatening bacterial infection.

The sponge should not be left inside the vagina for more than 30 hours. The sponge should not be used during menstruation or if you have a history of TSS.

Is a contraceptive sponge reversible?

Yes. The contraceptive sponge does not have any effects on either the male's or female's reproductive function. Pregnancy is possible when you stop using the contraceptive sponge.

What about a contraceptive sponge and sexually transmitted diseases (STDs)?

The contraceptive sponge does not provide protection against the transmission of sexually transmitted diseases.

What are the pros and cons of the contraceptive sponge?

The pros of the contraceptive sponge include:

- Easy to use and effective immediately

- Inexpensive

- Does not require a medical exam or prescription

- Reversible

The cons of the contraceptive sponge include:

- Does not protect against sexually transmitted diseases

- Side effects are rare

♣ It's A Fact!!

The contraceptive sponge is a soft, disk shaped device with a loop for removal. It is made out of polyurethane foam and contains the spermicide nonoxynol-9. Before intercourse, you wet the sponge and place it, loop side down, up inside your vagina to cover the cervix. The sponge is effective for more than one act of intercourse for up 24 hours. It needs to be left in for at least six hours after intercourse to prevent pregnancy and must be removed within 30 hours after it is inserted. Women who are sensitive to the spermicide nonoxynol-9 should not use this birth control method.

Source: Excerpted from "Birth Control Methods," The National Women's Health Information Center, U.S. Department of Health and Human Services, Office on Women's Health, July 2005.

Chapter 53

Oral Contraceptives

Why is this medication prescribed?

Oral contraceptives (birth control pills) are used to prevent pregnancy. Estrogen and progestin are two female sex hormones. Combinations of estrogen and progestin work by preventing ovulation (the release of eggs from the ovaries). They also change the lining of the uterus (womb) to prevent pregnancy from developing and change the mucus at the cervix (opening of the uterus) to prevent sperm (male reproductive cells) from entering. Oral contraceptives are a very effective method of birth control, but they do not prevent the spread of human immunodeficiency virus (HIV), the virus that causes acquired immunodeficiency syndrome (AIDS)) and other sexually transmitted diseases.

Some brands of oral contraceptives are also used to treat acne in certain patients. Oral contraceptives work to treat acne by decreasing the amounts of certain natural substances that can cause acne.

How should this medicine be used?

Oral contraceptives come in packets of 21, 28, or 91 tablets to take by mouth once a day, every day, or almost every day of a regular cycle. To avoid upset stomach, take oral contraceptives with food or milk. To help you remember to take your oral contraceptive regularly, take it at the same time every day (for example, after dinner or at bedtime). Follow the directions on your prescription label carefully and ask your doctor or pharmacist to explain any part you do not understand. Take your oral contraceptive exactly as directed. Do not take more or less of it, take it more often, or take it for a longer time than prescribed by your doctor.

If you have a 21-tablet packet, take one tablet daily for 21 days and then none for seven days. Then start a new packet.

✔ **Quick Tip**
Oral contraceptives come in many different brands. Different brands of oral contraceptives contain slightly different medications or doses, are taken in slightly different ways, and have different risks and benefits. Be sure that you know which brand of oral contraceptives you are using and exactly how you should use it. Ask your doctor or pharmacist for a copy of the manufacturer's information for the patient and read it carefully.

Source: © American Society of Health-System Pharmacists, Inc.

If you have a 28-tablet packet, take one tablet daily for 28 days. The last set of tablets are a different color. These tablets are reminder tablets. They do not contain any active ingredients, but taking one tablet every day will help you remember to start your next packet of birth control pills on time. The reminder tablets that come with certain brands of oral contraceptives contain iron. You should take one tablet daily continuously for 28 days in the order specified in your packet, starting a new packet the day after taking your 28th tablet.

If you have a 91-day tablet packet, take one tablet daily for 91 days. Your packet will contain three trays of tablets. Start with the first tablet on the first tray and continue taking one tablet every day in the order specified on the packet until you have taken all of the tablets on all of the trays. The last seven tablets are a different color. These tablets are not birth control pills; they contain an inactive ingredient. Start your new packet the day after you take your 91st tablet.

Your doctor will tell you when you should start taking your oral contraceptive. Oral contraceptives are usually started on the first or fifth day of your menstrual period or on the first Sunday after or on which bleeding begins. Your doctor will also tell you whether you need to use another method of birth control during the first seven days that you take your oral contraceptive and will help you choose a method. Follow these directions carefully.

Your menstrual period will probably begin while you are taking the inactive tablets, or during the week that you do not take your oral contraceptive, and may continue through that week. Be sure to start taking your new packet on schedule even if you are still bleeding.

You may need to use a backup method of birth control if you vomit or have diarrhea while you are taking an oral contraceptive. Talk to your doctor about this before you begin to take your oral contraceptive so that you can prepare a backup method of birth control in case it is needed. If you vomit or have diarrhea while you are taking an oral contraceptive, call your doctor to find out how long you should use the backup method.

If you have recently given birth, wait until four weeks after giving birth to begin taking oral contraceptives.

Oral contraceptives will work to prevent pregnancy or treat acne only as long as they are taken regularly. Continue to take oral contraceptives every day even if you are spotting or bleeding, have an upset stomach, or do not think that you are likely to become pregnant. Do not stop taking oral contraceptives without talking to your doctor.

What are other uses for this medicine?

Oral contraceptives are also sometimes used to treat heavy or irregular menstruation and endometriosis (a condition in which the type of tissue that lines the uterus [womb] grows in other areas of the body and causes pain, heavy or irregular menstruation [periods], and other symptoms). Talk to your doctor about the risks of using this medication for your condition.

What should I do if I forget a dose?

If you miss doses of your oral contraceptive, you may not be protected from pregnancy. You may need to use a backup method of birth control for seven days or until the end of the cycle. Every brand of oral contraceptives comes with specific directions to follow if you miss a dose. Carefully read the directions in the manufacturer's information for the patient that came with your oral contraceptive. If you have any questions, call your doctor or pharmacist. Continue to take your tablets as scheduled and use a backup method of birth control until your questions are answered.

What side effects can this medication cause?

Oral contraceptives may cause side effects. Tell your doctor if any of these symptoms are severe or do not go away:

- upset stomach
- vomiting
- stomach cramps or bloating
- diarrhea
- constipation
- gingivitis (swelling of the gum tissue)

- increased or decreased appetite
- weight gain or weight loss
- brown or black skin patches
- acne
- hair growth in unusual places
- bleeding or spotting between menstrual periods

♣ It's A Fact!!

First Contraceptive For Continuous Use

The U.S. Food and Drug Administration (FDA) has approved the first continuous-use drug product for the prevention of pregnancy. The contraceptive, Lybrel, is manufactured by Wyeth of Philadelphia, Pennsylvania.

Active Ingredients: Lybrel comes in a 28-day-pill pack with low-dose combination tablets that contain 90 micrograms of a progestin, levonorgestrel, and 20 micrograms of an estrogen, ethinyl estradiol. These are active ingredients available in other approved oral contraceptives.

How Lybrel Works: Continuous contraception works the same way as the 21-days-on/seven-days-off cycle. It stops the body's monthly preparation for pregnancy by lowering the production of hormones that make pregnancy possible. Other contraceptive pill regimens have placebo or pill-free intervals lasting four to seven days that stimulate a menstrual cycle. Lybrel is designed to be taken without the placebo or pill-free time interval. Women who use Lybrel would not have a scheduled menstrual period but will most likely have unplanned, breakthrough, unscheduled bleeding or spotting.

Unscheduled Bleeding Or Spotting: When considering the use of Lybrel, health professionals and patients should weigh the convenience of having no scheduled menstruation against the inconvenience of unscheduled bleeding or spotting. Unscheduled bleeding decreases over time in most women who continue to take Lybrel for a full year.

- changes in menstrual flow

- painful or missed periods

- breast tenderness, enlargement, or discharge

- difficulty wearing contact lenses

- swelling, redness, irritation, burning, or itching of the vagina

- white vaginal discharge

Some side effects can be serious. The following symptoms are uncommon, but if you experience any of them, call your doctor immediately:

- severe headache

- severe vomiting

Safety And Effectiveness: Like other available oral contraceptives, Lybrel is effective for pregnancy prevention when used as directed. The safety and effectiveness of Lybrel were supported by two one-year clinical studies, enrolling more than 2,400 women, ages 18 to 49. The risks of using Lybrel are similar to the risks of other conventional oral contraceptives.

- There is an increased risk of blood clots, heart attacks, and strokes.

- Cigarette smoking increases the risk of serious cardiovascular side effects from the use of combination estrogen and progestin-containing contraceptives.

- Because people who use Lybrel will not have regular periods, it may be difficult for women to recognize if they have become pregnant. Women should take a pregnancy test if they believe they may be pregnant.

- Birth control pills do not protect against human immunodeficiency virus/acquired immune deficiency syndrome (HIV/AIDS) or other sexually transmitted diseases.

Women should discuss contraceptive use, and the precautions and warnings for use of the drug product, with their doctor or other health care professional.

Source: Consumer Update, U.S. Food and Drug Administration, May 2007.

- speech problems

- dizziness or faintness

- weakness or numbness of an arm or leg

- crushing chest pain or chest heaviness

- coughing up blood

- shortness of breath

- pain, warmth, or heaviness in the back of the lower leg

- partial or complete loss of vision

- double vision

- bulging eyes

- severe stomach pain

- yellowing of the skin or eyes

- loss of appetite

- extreme tiredness, weakness, or lack of energy

- fever

- dark-colored urine

- light-colored stool

- swelling of the hands, feet, ankles, or lower legs

- depression, especially if you also have trouble sleeping, tiredness, loss of energy, or other mood changes

- unusual bleeding

- rash

Oral contraceptives may increase the chance that you will develop liver tumors. These tumors are not a form of cancer, but they can break and cause serious bleeding inside the body. Oral contraceptives may also increase the chance that you will develop breast or liver cancer, or have a heart attack, a stroke, or a serious blood clot. Talk to your doctor about the risks of using oral contraceptives.

Chapter 54

The Patch

The Basics

The patch—Ortho Evra—is a reversible prescription method of birth control. It is a thin, beige, plastic patch that sticks to the skin. A new patch is placed on the skin of the buttocks, stomach, upper outer arm, or upper torso once a week for three weeks in a row. No patch is used in the fourth week. The patch releases synthetic estrogen and progestin to protect against pregnancy for one month.

The hormones in the patch work by preventing a woman's ovaries from releasing eggs (ovulation). They also thicken the cervical mucus, which keeps sperm from joining with an egg. The hormones also thin the lining of the uterus. In theory, this could prevent pregnancy by interfering with implantation of a fertilized egg, but there is no scientific evidence that this occurs.

The patch works best when it is changed on the same day of the week for three weeks in a row. Pregnancy can happen if an error is made in using the patch—especially if:

- it becomes loose or falls off for more than 24 hours
- the same patch is left on the skin for more than one week

About This Chapter: "The Patch," reprinted with permission from Planned Parenthood® Federation of America, Inc. © 2007 PPFA. All rights reserved. For additional information, visit www.plannedparenthood.org.

If either of these things happens, follow the directions in your package insert, and call your clinician.

Effectiveness

The patch is a very effective reversible method of birth control. With typi-

> ## ✔ Quick Tip
> The patch does not protect against sexually transmitted infections. Always use a latex or female condom with the patch to reduce the risk of infection.

cal use, * although no studies have yet been published, it is assumed that the patch will be more effective than the pill—eight out of every 100 pill users become pregnant with typical use. Fewer than one woman out of every 100 women who use the patch will become pregnant with perfect use. **

The patch may be less effective for women who weigh more than 198 pounds.

Certain medicines and herbs may make the patch less effective. These include:

- the antibiotic rifampin. Other antibiotics do not make the patch less effective.
- certain anti-fungals that are taken orally for yeast infections
- certain anti-human immunodeficiency virus (HIV) protease inhibitors
- certain medicines used to treat seizures, mental illness, or headache
- St. John's wort

Talk to your clinician about the medicines you already take before you get a prescription for any method of birth control.

*Typical use refers to failure rates for women whose use is not consistent or always correct.

**Perfect use refers to failure rates for those whose use is consistent and always correct.

Advantages

The patch protects against pregnancy for one month. And it does not involve taking a daily pill.

Using the patch is simple, safe, and convenient.

Many women who use the patch have more regular, lighter, and shorter periods. And a woman's ability to become pregnant returns quickly when use of the patch is stopped.

The patch does not interfere with having sex, and may improve a woman's sex life. Some women say they feel free to be more spontaneous because they do not have to worry about becoming pregnant.

Results of long-term studies won't be available for some time, but researchers assume that the non-contraceptive advantages associated with the patch are similar to those known to be associated with the pill.

These health benefits may include some protection against:

- irregular menstrual cycles
- infection of the fallopian tubes (pelvic inflammatory disease), which often leads to infertility
- ectopic pregnancy (in the fallopian tubes)
- noncancerous breast growths
- ovarian cysts
- pelvic inflammatory disease, which often leads to infertility when left untreated
- cancer of the ovaries
- cancer of the lining of the uterus
- troublesome menstrual cramps
- iron deficiency anemia that results from heavy menses
- acne
- premenstrual symptoms, as well as related headaches and depression
- excess body hair
- osteoporosis—loss of bone mass
- vaginal dryness and painful intercourse associated with menopause

Possible Side Effects

As with all medications, there may be some undesirable side effects for some women taking combined hormone contraceptives. However, the patch is much safer than pregnancy and childbirth for healthy women—except among smokers age 35 and older.

Side effects that usually clear up after two or three months of use include:

• bleeding between periods

• breast tenderness

• changes in mood

• headache

• nausea—rarely, vomiting

Other possible side effects may include:

• change in sexual desire

• depression

• skin reaction at the site of application

Women with a history of depression may not be able to continue to use the patch if their depression worsens.

See your clinician right away if any problem develops while using the patch. Remember to tell any other clinician you may see that you are using the patch.

Possible Complications

Serious problems do not occur very often. In general, using the patch is much safer than pregnancy and childbirth. Combined-hormone contraception users have a slightly greater chance of certain major disorders than non-users. The risk is increased by being age 35 or older, smoking, and by having conditions associated with heart attack, such as diabetes, high blood pressure, or high cholesterol, and certain inherited conditions that increase the risk of blood clotting.

More estrogen is absorbed from the patch than from some other hormonal methods. The risks of heart attack, stroke, or blood clots in the lungs are rare for the patch, the pill, and the ring. There could be a slight increase in risk for blood clots in the legs for the patch users, but that hasn't been proven.

The most serious complication of combined-hormone use is having a blood clot in the legs, lungs, heart, or brain. Women on combined hormones who have major surgery or who have a leg immobilized—because they are confined to bed or have a cast—seem to have a greater chance of having blood clots. It is important to tell your surgeon that you are using the patch when planning a major operation. Follow your clinician's advice about when you can start using the patch again.

Rarely, women who use combined-hormone methods develop high blood pressure. Very rarely, they develop liver tumors, gallstones, or jaundice (yellowing of the skin or eyes).

Serious problems usually have warning signs. Report any of these signs to your clinician as soon as possible:

- Eye problems such as blurred or double vision

- Pain in the abdomen, chest, or arm

- Severe headaches

- Sudden shortness of breath or spitting up blood

- Unusual swelling or pain in the leg

- Worsening depression

- Yellowing of the skin or eyes (jaundice)

- A new lump in your breast

- Unusual heavy bleeding from your vagina

- No period after having a period every month

♣ **It's A Fact!!**
Combined-Hormone Contraception And Breast Cancer

The most recent research suggests that the use of combined-hormone methods has little, if any, effect on the risk of developing breast cancer.

Who Can Use The Patch

Most healthy women can use the patch. You should not use the patch if you:

- are 35 or older and smoke cigarettes
- have certain inherited blood clotting disorders
- have certain vascular conditions associated with diabetes mellitus
- have controlled high blood pressure and smoke cigarettes
- have had blood clots or vein inflammation
- have had an abnormal growth or cancer of the breast
- have had a heart attack or stroke
- have had migraine headaches with aura
- have had serious heart valve problems
- have a severe liver disease or have had growths on the liver
- have uncontrolled high blood pressure
- need prolonged bed rest after major surgery
- think you might be pregnant

Some patch users may need close medical supervision if they have:

- a body weight of 198 pounds or more
- diabetes—not associated with vascular conditions
- experienced jaundice (yellowing of the skin) during previous birth control use
- gallbladder disease
- high cholesterol or slightly increased blood pressure
- a high risk for heart disease
- a parent or sibling who has had a heart attack or stroke before age 55
- a seizure disorder that requires taking anticonvulsant medication
- unexplained bleeding from the vagina

Getting The Patch

Consult a clinician about using the patch. The clinician will discuss your medical history with you, check your blood pressure, and give any other medical exam that you may need. If the patch is right for you, the clinician will give you a prescription. Follow the instructions on the package.

You will place one new patch on the skin of the buttocks, stomach, upper outer arm, or upper torso once a week for three weeks in a row. You will not put on a patch for the fourth week.

- Store the patch at room temperature and keep it sealed until you apply it.
- Consider the first day you apply the patch as "patch change day."
- Gently tear the package along the top and side edges.
- Peel the foil pouch apart and open it flat. Then peel the patch and plastic layer off the foil liner.
- Next, peel half of the clear plastic away from the patch itself—do not touch the sticky part.
- Apply the sticky half of the patch to a clean and dry area of skin on the buttocks, stomach, upper outer arm, or upper torso—never on the breasts.
- Remove the other half of the plastic and press the full patch to the skin with your palm for ten seconds.
- Check your patch every day to make sure it is sticking in place.
- Remove it after one week. Reapply a new patch once a week on "patch change day" of the second and third weeks.
- After removal, fold the patch in half so that it sticks to itself, seal it in a plastic bag, and throw it out in the trash—do not flush.

During the one-week break, you will usually have your menstrual period. You may still be bleeding when it is time to apply a new patch. This is normal, too. But a new patch must be applied one week after the last one was removed—on "patch change day"—or pregnancy may occur.

If you apply your first patch within five days after the start of your period, you are protected immediately.

If you apply your first patch more than five days after the start of your period, use another method of birth control if you have vaginal intercourse during the first week— protection will begin after seven days.

What To Do If You Forget

If You Apply the Patch Late During Week One: Apply a new patch as soon as you remember. Use a backup method for seven days. Use emergency contraception if you have had unprotected vaginal intercourse. Change the patch one week after the day you applied your late patch—that will be your new "patch change day."

✔ Quick Tip
Where To Get The Patch And What It Costs

Visit Planned Parenthood, another family planning clinic, your health maintenance organization (HMO), or a private doctor for a prescription. The patch may be purchased at a drugstore or clinic.

Nationwide, the cost of an examination, if needed, ranges from about $35–$175. Costs vary from community to community, based on regional and local expenses. At some family planning clinics, the cost may depend on your income. The patch costs between $30 and $40 a month. The cost is usually lower at a clinic and is covered by Medicaid. Private health insurance coverage for birth control varies.

If You Apply the Patch Late During Week Two or Three: If you are one or two days late changing your patch, change it as soon as you remember. Maintain your regular "patch change day" for the next patch.

If you are more than two days late changing your patch, change it as soon as you remember. This will be your new "patch change day." Use a backup method for seven days. Use emergency contraception if you have had unprotected vaginal intercourse. Wear the late patch for one week.

If You Apply the Patch Late During Week Four: Remove the patch. Apply a new patch on your regular "patch change day."

If a patch becomes loose or falls off:

- for less than one day, reapply the patch. If the patch will not stick well, apply a new patch. Change the patch on your regular "patch change day."

- for more than one day, or if you are unsure how long it has been loose or off, apply a new patch. This will be your new "patch change day." Use a backup method for seven days. Use emergency contraception if you have had unprotected vaginal intercourse. Wear the replacement patch for one week.

Pregnancy And The Patch

There is a very slight chance that you will become pregnant even if you use the patch.

However, a missed period does not always mean you are pregnant, especially if you have used the patch correctly. But see your clinician if you miss a second period.

It is unlikely that using the patch during early pregnancy will increase the risk of defects in the fetus.

If you want to become pregnant, stop using the patch. If you want to plan the timing of your pregnancy, use another form of birth control until your period becomes regular. It usually takes about one to three months for your period to return to the cycle you had before using the patch.

Starting The Patch After Pregnancy

After childbirth, wait at least two weeks before applying the patch. Use a backup method for seven days if you have not yet gotten your period.

The patch may reduce the amount and quality of milk in the first six weeks of breastfeeding. Also, the milk will contain traces of the patch's hormones. If you are breastfeeding, wait at least six weeks after childbirth to apply the patch. Use a backup method for seven days if you have not yet gotten your period.

You can start using the patch immediately after having an abortion. Use a backup method of birth control for seven days if you start the patch:

• more than five days after a vacuum aspiration abortion

• more than seven days after taking mifepristone

Chapter 55

The Shot

Depo-Provera is an injection of a hormone called progestin. It is similar to the body's natural hormone progesterone. Depo-Provera injections prevent a woman's ovaries from releasing eggs. Depo-Provera is more than 99 percent effective and is generally considered the most effective reversible method of birth control. Used alone, it doesn't protect you against sexually transmitted infections.

How Depo-Provera Is Administered

Injections of Depo-Provera are given every 12 weeks to prevent pregnancy. You can get these shots from a doctor or clinic. Women who have a Depo-Provera injection must not be pregnant at the time of the first injection. To avoid this, it is best to have the first injection:

- in the first five days of your menstrual period
- within five days of an abortion
- within five days of giving birth

If you do not have the injection at one of these times, you should use another method of birth control as back-up for two full weeks so you don't get pregnant. Depo-Provera is safe when you are breast-feeding.

About This Chapter: Information in this chapter is from "Depo-Provera Injections." Reprinted with permission from www.womenshealthmatters.ca. © 2000–2007. Women's College Hospital.

Most women have some irregularities in the menstrual bleeding after starting Depo-Provera injections. Periods often stop altogether after six to twelve months using Depo-Provera. The effects of Depo-Provera can last for some time after you choose to stop the injections, as it takes some time for the hormone to clear out of your system. While most women get their periods within six months of their last injection, some women take up to two years to get their periods back.

Advantages

- Women who have health conditions that prevent them from taking birth control pills can often take Depo-Provera.

- Very effective at preventing pregnancy

- You don't have to interrupt sex.

- The woman controls this method of birth control.

- You don't have to remember a daily pill.

- Very safe

Disadvantages

- You are not protected against sexually transmitted infections.

♣ **It's A Fact!!**
Large studies have not shown any link between Depo-Provera use and breast cancer, but research is still being done in this area. Researchers are also studying whether Depo-Provera can decrease a woman's bone mineral density, increasing her risk of osteoporosis.

- You may have irregular menstrual bleeding or more frequent bleeding.

- You must return to the clinic/doctor every 12 weeks for your injection.

- You may experience side effects (see below).

- Women with some medical conditions cannot use Depo-Provera. (Women should not use this method if they have abnormal vaginal bleeding, liver diseases such as jaundice or hepatitis, or breast cancer.)

- While unlikely, you may not be able to get pregnant for up to two years after using Depo-Provera.

Side Effects

Some women who use Depo-Provera experience side effects. If these side effects interfere with your life, you may wish to consider other methods of birth control. Women on Depo-Provera may experience:

- irregular menstrual bleeding or more frequent periods (Most women have no periods at all after 6–12 months.)

- weight gain of more than two pounds each year when Depo-Provera is used (This weight gain may continue for a number of months after you stop using Depo-Provera.)

- headaches

- breast tenderness

- bloating

- depression

- unwanted hair or hair loss

Chapter 56

Intrauterine Devices And Systems

Intrauterine devices include plastic and copper devices (IUD) and hormone releasing devices called intrauterine systems (IUS).

What Is An IUD?

An IUD is a small plastic and copper device, which is inserted into your uterus (womb) by a doctor to prevent pregnancy. IUDs come in different shapes and sizes.

What Is An IUS?

The IUS (brand name Mirena) is a plastic device similar to the IUD but contains a progestogen hormone called levonorgestrel.

How Do They Work?

Copper IUDs primarily work by affecting sperm movement, stopping them from moving through the uterus. They also cause changes to the lining of the uterus (endometrium), which in the rare instance of an egg being fertilized, prevent the egg from attaching to the endometrium. The IUD is sometimes used as a form of emergency contraception up to the fifth day after unprotected intercourse.

About This Chapter: Information in this chapter is from "Intrauterine Devices and Systems," © 2006 Family Planning Association of Western Australia (www.fpwa.au). All rights reserved. Reprinted with permission.

Progestogen IUSs work by releasing a progestogen hormone at a steady rate, thinning the lining of the uterus and making it difficult for an egg to implant or for sperm to move towards the egg.

How Effective Are They?

IUDs and IUSs are more than 99 percent effective at preventing pregnancy. Copper IUDs are effective for five to eight years, depending on the type. IUDs inserted in women over the age of 40 can be left until after menopause. Progestogen IUSs provide effective contraception for five years, after which time they need changing.

Who Can Use An IUD Or IUS?

IUDs and IUSs are effective, safe, and reliable long-term methods of contraception for many women. Your doctor will take a detailed medical history to ensure that an IUD or IUS is suitable for you.

A copper IUD or progestogen IUS is not suitable for a woman who:

- has a pelvic infection
- is or could be pregnant (though an IUD can be used as emergency contraception)
- has abnormal vaginal bleeding for which the cause has not been found
- has a high risk of acquiring a sexually transmissible infection (STI)

Copper IUDs are also not suitable for women who have very heavy, painful, or prolonged periods, or who have iron deficiency anemia.

A copper IUD or progestogen IUS may not be suitable for a woman who has:

- never had a child
- more than one sexual partner, or a partner who has other partners
- a bleeding disorder
- valvular heart disease
- a uterine abnormality such as fibroids

When Can An IUD Or IUS Be Inserted?

A copper IUD can be inserted at any time in your cycle if pregnancy can confidently be excluded. For this reason, the device is usually put in between the first day of your period and ovulation.

A progestogen IUS can only be inserted between day one (first day of menstrual bleeding) to day seven of the menstrual cycle.

How Is It Done?

The insertion of an IUD or IUS does not require a general anesthetic. The doctor will do an internal examination to determine the size and position of your uterus. A speculum is put into your vagina so that the doctor can see the cervix. After measuring the length of the uterus with a small metal rod, the device is inserted. Many women have cramping similar to period pain, but this usually wears off very quickly.

Some women may feel faint, but again, will recover quickly. Women who have not had children may experience more pain or discomfort when the device is inserted.

What To Do After Your IUD Or IUS Is Inserted

It is recommended that women don't put anything into their vagina for 48 hours after the insertion of an IUD or IUS to reduce the risk of infection. This means no tampons (use pads), no intercourse, no swimming, and no baths (shower instead) for two days after insertion.

✔ **Quick Tip**
It is recommended that women be screened for genital infections prior to the insertion of an IUD or IUS. If a Pap smear is due, this can be done at the same time.

You will need to visit your doctor for a checkup after your next period and then once each year. Every second year this can coincide with your Pap smear.

In a small percentage of women, the IUD or IUS can be expelled by the uterus. This most commonly happens in the first month after insertion. Expulsion is more common in women who have never had children.

Learn to check the thread of your IUD or IUS. This tells you that it is still in place and has not been expelled by your uterus, perhaps during a period. Most pregnancies that occur in women using IUDs and IUSs are due to unnoticed expulsion.

To feel the thread, place two fingers deep in your vagina and feel for the firm knob (like the end of your nose) that is your cervix. The thread should come out of the cervix and lie next to it.

You should check the thread once a month after your period before you rely on it for contraception. Many women find this convenient to do in the shower. If you cannot feel the thread (and it can be hard to find), go back to the clinic for a checkup, and use other contraception until then.

Advantages

Copper IUDs and progestogen IUSs:

- are very effective and safe forms of long term contraception

- are cheap considering how long they last

- do not usually interfere with your normal hormonal cycle

- are a suitable method of contraception for some women who are unable to take the pill

- can be removed at any time, and fertility returns quickly

- do not have any metabolic effects (for example, cholesterol and blood clotting)

Unlike copper IUDs, progestogen IUSs are suitable for women who have heavy menstrual bleeding. Women using an IUS often have lighter, less painful periods, or none at all.

Aside from its use as a contraceptive device, progestogen IUSs can also be used as an alternative to surgical or oral hormonal treatments for women with heavy menstrual bleeding, and by menopausal women taking oestrogen who cannot tolerate other forms of progestogen.

Disadvantages

Periods may be heavier, longer, and more painful with a copper IUD. This often settles after the first few months.

After having a progestogen IUS inserted, some women experience frequent (but light) bleeding in the first few months. Some also experience hormonal side effects, such as mood changes or breast tenderness.

Possible Risks

Pelvic Infection

The risk of pelvic infection is highest in the first few weeks following insertion. Screening is recommended for vaginal and cervical infections prior to insertion to reduce the risk of these infections being passed into the uterus. After these first few weeks, the risk of pelvic infection is no greater than normal in a woman using an IUD or IUS unless she changes partners, has more than one sexual partner, or her partner has more than one sexual partner (that is, her partner has an STI). A pelvic infection may cause damage to the fallopian tubes, which can lead to infertility. It can also cause chronic pelvic pain. Possible symptoms of infection include:

- pain or tenderness in the lower abdomen
- unusual bleeding from the vagina
- fever or chills
- discharge from the vagina
- deep pain during intercourse
- a burning sensation when passing urine

Pregnancy With An IUD Or IUS In Place

Modern IUDs and IUSs are now more than 99 percent effective. In other words, less than 1 out of every 100 women using them for a year will get pregnant. If you have an IUD or IUS and think you may be pregnant, see your doctor to get it removed. If the device is left in position during pregnancy, there is a higher risk of miscarriage later in the pregnancy. Of those rare pregnancies that may occur with an IUD or IUS, a slightly greater proportion may be an ectopic pregnancy (pregnancy in fallopian tube). For this reason, if you feel you might be pregnant, it is very important to see your doctor.

Perforation

In a small number of cases (1–2 per thousand insertions), the IUD or IUS may be pushed through the wall of the uterus and then require removal by an operation. This risk is reduced if the doctor fitting the IUD or IUS is very skilled in insertion.

Short Wave Diathermy Treatment

Women with copper IUDs should not have short wave diathermy treatment to the abdomen or lower back. Diathermy is used by physiotherapists in the treatment of some kinds of muscular pain. IUDs and IUSs do not cause problems with other treatment such as ultrasound or massage. If in doubt, tell the treating doctor that you have an IUD in place.

Removal

Never attempt this yourself. A doctor will remove the IUD or IUS at your request. Cramping and some bleeding may be experienced when the device is removed.

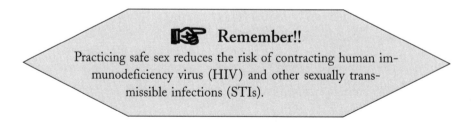

☞ Remember!!
Practicing safe sex reduces the risk of contracting human immunodeficiency virus (HIV) and other sexually transmissible infections (STIs).

Chapter 57

Vaginal Ring

Etonogestrel and ethinyl estradiol vaginal ring is used to prevent pregnancy. Etonogestrel and ethinyl estradiol vaginal ring is in a class of medications called combination hormonal contraceptives (birth control medications). Etonogestrel is a progestin and ethinyl estradiol is an estrogen. Etonogestrel and ethinyl estradiol vaginal ring works by preventing ovulation (the release of an egg from the ovaries). It also changes the lining of the uterus (womb) to prevent pregnancy from developing and changes the mucus at the cervix (opening of the uterus) to prevent sperm (male reproductive cells) from entering.

How should the vaginal ring be used?

Etonogestrel and ethinyl estradiol combination comes as a flexible ring to place in the vagina. It is usually placed in the vagina and left in place for three weeks. After three weeks, it is removed for a one-week break; then a new ring is inserted. Follow the directions on your prescription label carefully and ask your doctor or pharmacist to explain any part you do not understand. Use the contraceptive ring exactly as directed. Never use more than one contraceptive ring at a time and always insert and remove the ring according to the schedule your doctor gives you.

You should always insert and remove the contraceptive ring on the same day of the week and at about the same time of day. Your menstrual period will probably start two to three days after you remove the contraceptive ring and may continue through that week. Be sure to insert your new ring at the end of the week on the same day and at the same time that you usually insert or remove the ring even if you have not stopped bleeding.

♣ **It's A Fact!!**
The contraceptive ring is a very effective method of birth control but does not prevent the spread of human immunodeficiency virus (HIV), the virus that causes acquired immunodeficiency syndrome (AIDS) or other sexually transmitted diseases.

Your doctor will tell you when you should insert your first contraceptive ring. This depends on whether you were using a different type of birth control in the past month, were not using birth control, or have recently given birth, or had an abortion or miscarriage. In some cases, you may need to use an additional method of birth control for the first seven days that you use the contraceptive ring. Your doctor will tell you whether you need to use backup birth control and will help you choose a method, such as male condoms and/or spermicides. You should not use a diaphragm when a contraceptive ring is in place.

You do not need to position the contraceptive ring a certain way inside your vagina. The ring will work no matter how it is positioned but will be more comfortable and less likely to fall out when it is placed as far back in your vagina as possible. The ring cannot get past the cervix, so it will not go too far into the vagina or get lost when you push it in.

The contraceptive ring will usually stay in your vagina until you remove it. It may sometimes slip out when you are removing a tampon or having a bowel movement, or if you are very constipated or have not placed it properly in your vagina. Call your doctor if your contraceptive ring slips out often.

If your contraceptive ring slips out, you should rinse it with cool or lukewarm (not hot) water and replace it in your vagina as soon as possible. If your ring gets lost, you should replace it with a new ring and remove the new ring at the same time you were scheduled to remove the ring that was lost. Try to replace your ring within three hours after it falls out. If you do not replace your ring within three hours, you must use a backup method of birth control until you have had the ring in place for seven days in a row.

To use the contraceptive ring, follow these steps:

- Wash and dry your hands.

- Remove one contraceptive ring from its foil pouch, but do not throw away the pouch. Put the pouch in a safe place so you can use it to properly throw away the contraceptive ring after you remove it.

- Lie down on your back with your knees bent, squat, or stand with one leg up on a chair, step, or other object. Choose the position that is most comfortable for you.

- Hold the contraceptive ring between your thumb and index finger and press the opposite sides of the ring together.

- Gently push the folded ring into your vagina.

- If you feel discomfort, push the ring further back into your vagina with your index finger.

- Wash your hands again.

- When it is time to remove the contraceptive ring, hook your index finger under the front rim or hold the rim between your index and middle fingers and pull it out.

- Put the used ring into the foil pouch and throw it away in a trash can that is out of the reach of children and pets. Do not throw the used ring in the toilet.

- Wash your hands.

- Wait one week, and then insert a new ring following the directions above.

What special precautions should I follow?

Before using etonogestrel and ethinyl estradiol vaginal ring, do the following:

- Tell your doctor and pharmacist if you are allergic to etonogestrel, ethinyl estradiol, or any other medications.

- Tell your doctor and pharmacist what other prescription and nonprescription medications, vitamins, and nutritional supplements you are taking. Your doctor may need to change the doses of your medications or monitor you carefully for side effects. You may need to use an extra method of birth control if you take certain medications while you are using the contraceptive ring.

- Tell your doctor what herbal products you are taking, especially products containing St. John's wort.

- Tell your doctor if you have or have ever had, or anyone in your family has or has ever had, breast cancer, if you have ever had yellowing of the skin or eyes during pregnancy or while you were using another type of hormonal contraceptive (birth control pills, patches, rings, or injections), if you are on bed rest or are unable to walk around for any reason, or if you have or have ever had breast lumps; an abnormal mammogram (breast x-ray); fibrocystic breast disease (swollen, tender breasts and/or breast lumps that are not cancer); any type of cancer, especially cancer of the endometrium (lining of the uterus), cervix, or vagina; blood clots in your legs, lungs, or eyes; stroke or mini-stroke; coronary artery disease (clogged blood vessels leading to the heart); chest pain; a heart attack; any condition that affects your heart valves (flaps of tissue that open and close to control blood flow in the heart); high cholesterol or triglycerides; high blood pressure; diabetes; headaches; seizures; depression; unexplained vaginal bleeding; any condition that makes your vagina more likely to become irritated; bladder, uterus or rectum that has dropped or bulged into the vagina; constipation; or liver, kidney, thyroid, or gallbladder disease.

- Tell your doctor if you are pregnant or plan to become pregnant. If you become pregnant while using etonogestrel and ethinyl estradiol vaginal ring, call your doctor immediately. You should suspect that you are pregnant and call your doctor if you have used the contraceptive ring correctly and you miss two periods in a row, or if you have not used the contraceptive ring according to the directions and you miss one period. You should not breastfeed while you are using the contraceptive ring.

- If you are having surgery, including dental surgery, tell the doctor or dentist that you are using etonogestrel and ethinyl estradiol vaginal ring.

- Tell your doctor if you wear contact lenses. If you notice changes in your vision or your ability to wear your lenses while using etonogestrel and ethinyl estradiol vaginal ring, see an eye doctor.

♣ It's A Fact!!

Cigarette smoking increases the risk of serious side effects from etonogestrel and ethinyl estradiol vaginal ring, including heart attacks, blood clots, and strokes. This risk is higher for women over 35 years old and heavy smokers (15 or more cigarettes per day). If you use etonogestrel and ethinyl estradiol ring, you should not smoke.

What special dietary instructions should I follow?

Talk to your doctor about drinking grapefruit juice while using the vaginal ring.

What should I do if I forget a dose?

If you forget to insert a new contraceptive ring one week after you removed the old ring, you may not be protected from pregnancy. Check to be sure that you are not pregnant. If you are not pregnant, insert a new ring as soon as you remember and use a backup method of birth control until the new ring has been in place for seven days in a row.

If you forget to remove the contraceptive ring on time but remember before one week has passed, remove the ring as soon as you remember. Wait one week and then insert a new ring. If you forget to remove the contraceptive ring and remember after more than one week has passed, you may not be protected from pregnancy. Check to be sure that you are not pregnant. If you are not pregnant, remove the ring as soon as you remember, wait one week and insert a new ring. Use a backup method of birth control until the new ring has been in place for seven days in a row.

What side effects can the vaginal ring cause?

Etonogestrel and ethinyl estradiol vaginal ring may cause side effects. Tell your doctor if any of these symptoms are severe or do not go away:

- swelling, redness, irritation, burning, itching, or infection of the vagina
- white or yellow vaginal discharge
- vaginal bleeding or spotting when it is not time for your period. (Call your doctor if the bleeding lasts longer than a few days or happens in more than one cycle.)
- headache
- runny nose
- upset stomach
- vomiting
- changes in appetite
- weight gain or loss
- stomach cramps or bloating
- nervousness
- breasts that are large, tender, or produce a liquid
- growth of hair on face
- loss of hair on scalp
- acne
- changes in sexual desire

Some side effects can be serious. The following symptoms are uncommon, but if you experience any of them call your doctor immediately:

- pain in the back of the lower leg

- sharp, sudden, or crushing chest pain

- heaviness in chest

- coughing up blood

- sudden shortness of breath

- sudden severe headache, vomiting, dizziness, or fainting

- sudden problems with speech

- weakness or numbness of an arm or leg

- sudden loss of vision

- double vision, blurred vision, or other changes in vision

- bulging eyes

- yellowing of the skin or eyes, especially if you also have fever, tiredness, loss of appetite, dark urine, and/or light-colored bowel movements

- depression, especially if you also have trouble sleeping, tiredness, loss of energy, or other mood changes

- pain, tenderness, or swelling of the abdomen (area between the chest and the waist)

- stomach pain that worsens after eating

- swelling of the hands, feet, ankles, or lower legs

- diarrhea

- painful, difficult, or frequent urination

- brown patches on the skin, especially the face

- rash

Etonogestrel and ethinyl estradiol vaginal ring may increase the chance that you will develop liver tumors. These tumors are not a form of cancer, but they can break and cause serious bleeding inside the body. The contraceptive ring may also increase the chance that you will develop breast or liver cancer, or have a heart attack, a stroke, or a serious blood clot. Talk to your doctor about the risks of using the contraceptive ring.

Etonogestrel and ethinyl estradiol vaginal ring may cause other side effects. Call your doctor if you have any unusual problems while using the vaginal ring.

What storage conditions are needed for the vaginal ring?

Keep it in the packet it came in, tightly closed, and out of reach of children. Store it at room temperature and away from excess heat and moisture (not in the bathroom). Throw away any vaginal rings that are outdated or no longer needed. Talk to your pharmacist about proper disposal.

Can an overdose occur?

Etonogestrel and ethinyl estradiol vaginal ring is unlikely to cause an overdose. You will not receive too much medication if the ring breaks inside your vagina or if it is left in your vagina for too long.

Symptoms of overdose may include the following:

- upset stomach
- vomiting
- vaginal bleeding
- irregular period

☞ **Remember!!**
Before having any laboratory test, tell your doctor and the laboratory personnel that you are using etonogestrel and ethinyl estradiol vaginal ring.

Chapter 58

Sterilization

Tubal Ligation

Tubal ligation is an operation, which blocks the tubes carrying a woman's egg to her uterus. Worldwide, it is the most commonly used method of birth control. Often the operation is performed through a laparoscope. This instrument is inserted through a small incision in the abdomen. The tubes are visualized so the surgeon can place rings on, or apply clips to, the tubes or burn the tubes.

After a tubal sterilization the egg cannot reach the uterus, and the man's sperm cannot reach the egg. This operation should be considered permanent. You must be certain you do not want to deliver more children and will not change your mind. Complete information about this surgical procedure is available from your clinician.

Advantages

- Tubal sterilization is an effective contraceptive when no more children are desired.

About This Chapter: Information under the heading "Tubal Ligation" is reprinted from the Family Planning Program, Department of Gynecology and Obstetrics, Emory University School of Medicine, www.gynob.emory.edu/familyplanning. Text under the heading "Vasectomy," is excerpted from "Facts About Vasectomy Safety," National Institute of Child Health and Human Development, National Institutes of Health, August 2006.

- It is a fairly simple operation, which is safe and permanent.

- Nothing must be taken daily or used at the time of sexual intercourse.

- Tubal sterilization will not affect your sex drive or ability to enjoy sex.

- It is cost-effective in the long run.

Disadvantages

- Tubal sterilization requires minor surgery (an operation).

- There may be some pain or discomfort for several days after the operation.

- You must have someone accompany you on the day of the surgery.

- There is no easy way to check after tubal sterilization to see if it is "still working."

- Tubal sterilization is very effective but not 100% effective. The failure rate is 1–5% during the first ten years after the operation. If you think that you are pregnant after having a tubal sterilization, return to the clinic immediately. Should a pregnancy occur, there is an increased chance that the pregnancy will be outside of your uterus (an ectopic pregnancy).

- It is difficult to reverse this operation if you want to become pregnant at a later time. The operation to reverse tubal sterilization is highly technical, expensive, and its results cannot be guaranteed.

- Regret after tubal sterilization is greater if a woman is under 25 when her operation is done, if she divorces or remarries, if a child dies, or if a woman has just had a baby or an abortion when she has her operation.

- Sterilization will not protect you from human immunodeficiency virus (HIV) or other infections. Use a condom if you or your partner may be at risk.

- In most states a consent form and a 30-day waiting period are required before scheduling the procedure.

Where Can I Go To Get This Operation?

You can get a referral to a clinician who does the tubal sterilization operation from your primary care provider, health department, family planning clinic, or local medical society.

Vasectomy

Vasectomy is a simple operation designed to make a man sterile, or unable to father a child. It is used as a means of contraception in many parts of the world. A total of about 50 million men have had a vasectomy—a number that corresponds to roughly 5 percent of all married couples of reproductive age. In comparison, about 15 percent of couples rely on female sterilization for birth control.

Approximately half a million vasectomies are performed in the United States each year. About one out of six men over age 35 has been vasectomized, the prevalence increasing along with education and income. Among married couples in this country, only female sterilization and oral contraception are relied upon more often for family planning.

Vasectomy involves blocking the tubes through which sperm pass into the semen. Sperm are produced in a man's testis and stored in an adjacent structure known as the epididymis. During sexual climax, the sperm move from the epididymis through a tube called the vas deferens and mix with other components of semen to form the ejaculate. All vasectomy techniques involve cutting or otherwise blocking both the left and right vas deferens, so the man's ejaculate will no longer contain sperm, and he will not be able to make a woman pregnant.

Vasectomy Techniques

In the conventional approach, a physician makes one or two small incisions, or cuts, in the skin of the scrotum, which has been numbed with a local anesthetic. The vas is cut, and a small piece may be removed. Next, the doctor ties the cut ends and sews up the scrotal incision. The entire procedure is then repeated on the other side.

An improved method, devised by a Chinese surgeon, has been widely used in China since 1974. This so-called non-surgical or no-scalpel vasectomy was introduced into the United States in 1988, and many doctors are now using the technique here.

In a no-scalpel vasectomy, the doctor feels for the vas under the skin of the scrotum and holds it in place with a small clamp. Then a special instrument is used to make a tiny puncture in the skin and stretches the opening so the vas can be cut and tied. This approach produces very little bleeding, and no stitches are needed to close the punctures, which heal quickly by themselves. The newer method also produces less pain and fewer complications than conventional vasectomy.

Post-Vasectomy

Regardless of how it is performed, vasectomy offers many advantages as a method of birth control. Like female sterilization, it is a highly effective one-time procedure that provides permanent contraception. But vasectomy is medically much simpler than female sterilization, has a lower incidence of complications, and is much less expensive.

After vasectomy, the patient will probably feel sore for a few days, and he should rest for at least one day. However, he can expect to recover completely in less than a week. Many men have the procedure on a Friday and return to work on Monday. Although complications such as swelling, bruising, inflammation, and infection may occur, they are relatively uncommon and almost never serious. Nevertheless, men who develop these symptoms at any time should inform their physician.

A man can resume sexual activity within a few days after vasectomy, but precautions should be taken against pregnancy until a test shows that his semen is free of sperm. Generally, this test is performed after the patient has had 10–20 post-vasectomy ejaculations. If sperm are still present in the semen, the patient is told to return later for a repeat test.

A major study of vasectomy side effects occurring within 8 to 10 years after the procedure was published in the *British Medical Journal* in 1992. The National Institute of Child Health and Human Development (NICHD) sponsored this study, the Health Status of American Men, or HSAM. Investigators questioned 10,590 vasectomized men, and an equal number of non-vasectomized men, to see if they had developed any of 99 different disorders. After a total of 182,000 person-years of follow-up, only one condition, epididymitis/orchitis (defined as painful, swollen, and tender epididymis or testis), was found to be more common after vasectomy. This local inflammation most often occurs during the first year after surgery. Treated with heat, it usually clears up within a week.

Disadvantages Of Vasectomy

The chief advantage of vasectomy, its permanence, is also its chief disadvantage. The procedure itself is simple, but reversing it is difficult, expensive, and often unsuccessful. Researchers are studying new methods of blocking the vas that may produce less tissue damage and scarring and might thus permit more successful reversal. But these methods are all experimental, and their effectiveness has not yet been confirmed. It is possible to store semen in a sperm bank to preserve the possibility of producing a pregnancy at some future date. However, doing this is costly, and the sperm in stored semen do not always remain viable (able to cause pregnancy). For all of these reasons, doctors advise that only men who are prepared to accept the fact that they will no longer be able to father a child undertake vasectomy. The decision should be considered along with other contraceptive options and discussed with a professional counselor. Men who are married, or in a serious relationship, should also discuss the issue with their partners.

♣ It's A Fact!!

Although it is extremely effective for preventing pregnancy, vasectomy does not offer protection against AIDS or other sexually transmitted diseases. Consequently, it is important that vasectomized men continue to use condoms, preferably latex, which offer considerable protection against the spread of disease, in any sexual encounter that carries the risk of contracting or transmitting infection.

Source: National Institute of Child Health
and Human Development

Masculinity And Sexuality

Vasectomy does not affect production or release of testosterone, the male hormone responsible for a man's sex drive, beard, deep voice, and other masculine traits. The operation also has no effect on sexuality. Erections, climaxes, and the amount of ejaculate remain the same.

Occasionally, a man may experience sexual difficulties after vasectomy, but these almost always have an emotional basis and can usually be alleviated with counseling. More often, men who have undergone the procedure, and their partners, find that sex is more spontaneous and enjoyable once they are freed from concerns about contraception and accidental pregnancy.

✎ What's It Mean?

Tubal Ligation: An operation to tie the fallopian tubes closed. This procedure prevents pregnancy by blocking the passage of eggs from the ovaries to the uterus.

Vasectomy: An operation to cut or tie off the two tubes that carry sperm out of the testicles.

Source: "Dictionary of Cancer Terms," National Cancer Institute, U.S. National Institutes of Health; cited August 2007.

Chapter 59

Emergency Contraception

What is emergency contraception (or emergency birth control)?

Emergency contraception, or emergency birth control, is used to help keep a woman from getting pregnant after she has had unprotected sex (sex without using birth control).

Use emergency contraception in the following situations:

• You did not use birth control.

• You were forced to have sex.

• The condom broke or came off.

• He did not pull out in time.

• You missed two or more birth control pills in a row.

• You were late getting your shot.

Emergency contraception should not be used as regular birth control. Other birth control methods are much better at keeping women from becoming pregnant. Talk with your doctor to decide which one is right for you.

About This Chapter: The National Women's Health Information Center, U.S. Department of Health and Human Services, Office on Women's Health, May 2006.

How does emergency contraception work?

Emergency contraception can keep you from becoming pregnant by doing one of the following:

- Keeping the egg from leaving the ovary
- Keeping the sperm from meeting the egg
- Keeping the fertilized egg from attaching to the uterus (womb)

If you are already pregnant, emergency contraception will not work.

What are the types of emergency contraception?

There are two types. They are as follows:

- Emergency contraceptive pills (ECPs)
- Intrauterine devices (IUDs)

ECPs contain higher doses of the same hormones in some brands of regular birth control pills. Some ECPs are "combined ECPs" with progestin and estrogen. Others are progestin-only. If you are breastfeeding, or if you cannot take estrogen, you should use progestin-only ECPs. You should always take ECPs as soon as you can after having sex, but they can work up to five days later. The two types of ECPs are as follows:

- **Plan B (Progestin-Only):** Made for use as emergency contraception. The two pills can be taken in two doses (one pill right away and the next pill 12 hours later), or both pills can be taken at the same time. Some women feel sick and throw up after taking ECPs. Taking both pills at the same time will not increase your chances of having these side effects. If you throw up after taking ECPs, call your doctor or pharmacist.

- **Higher Dose of Regular Birth Control Pills:** The number of pills in a dose is different for each pill brand, and not all brands can be used for emergency contraception. For more information on birth control pills that can be used for emergency contraception, visit Not-2-Late.com. The pills are taken in two doses (one dose right away and the next dose 12 hours later). Always use the same brand for both doses. Some women feel sick and throw up after taking ECPs. If you throw up after taking ECPs, call your doctor or pharmacist.

The other type of emergency contraception is the IUD. The IUD is a T-shaped plastic device placed into the uterus (womb) by a doctor within five days after having sex.

The IUD works by doing one of the following:

- Keeping the sperm from meeting the egg
- Keeping the egg from attaching to the uterus (womb)

Your doctor can remove the IUD after your next period, or it can be left in place for up to ten years to use as your regular birth control.

Are emergency contraceptive pills (ECPs) the same thing as the "morning after pill"?

Yes. ECPs are often called the "morning after pill," which is wrong because ECPs are never taken as only one pill and they do not have to be taken the morning after. You should always take ECPs as soon as you can after having unprotected sex (sex without using birth control), but they can work up to five days later.

How do I get emergency contraceptive pills (ECPs)?

Plan B (progestin-only) was recently approved to be sold over-the-counter to women who are 18 years of age or older. Women under the age of 18 will need a prescription. Women will have to show proof of age to buy Plan B.

Can I get emergency contraceptive pills (ECPs) before I need them?

Yes. Your doctor should bring up ECPs at your annual exam (when you have a pap smear or pap test). If your doctor does not talk about emergency contraception at your next exam, ask for it.

Will ECPs protect me from sexually transmitted diseases (STDs)?

No. ECPs can only keep you from becoming pregnant. Always use condoms to lower your risk of getting a sexually transmitted disease.

What do I need to do after I take emergency contraceptive pills (ECPs)?

Take the ECPs exactly as your doctor or pharmacist tells you to. If you see another doctor or nurse for any reason after taking ECPs, tell him/her that you have taken ECPs.

Some women feel sick and throw up after taking ECPs. This side effect happens more often with pills that contain both estrogen and progestin. Your doctor or pharmacist can give you medication to help control sickness. If you throw up after taking ECPs, call your doctor or pharmacist. After you have taken ECPs, your next period may come sooner or later than normal. Your period also may be heavier, lighter, or more spotty than normal. Use another birth control method if you have sex any time before your next period starts.

If you do not get your period in three weeks, or if you think you might be pregnant after taking ECPs, consider getting a pregnancy test just to make sure you are not pregnant.

Does emergency contraception work all the time?

No. Emergency contraceptive pills (ECPs) that contain both estrogen and progestin are about 75 percent effective at keeping a woman from getting pregnant. In other words, if 100 women had unprotected sex (sex without using birth control) in the fertile part of their cycle (when an egg is most likely to leave the ovary), about eight of those women would become pregnant. If all 100 women took combined emergency contraceptive pills, only two would become pregnant. ECPs containing only progestin are about 89 percent effective. If those same 100 women took progestin-only ECPs, only one would become pregnant. The IUD is 99.9 percent effective. If 1,000 women had an IUD put in, only one would become pregnant.

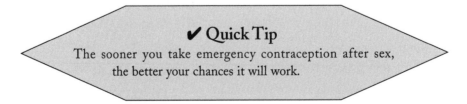

✔ Quick Tip

The sooner you take emergency contraception after sex, the better your chances it will work.

My girlfriend took emergency contraceptive pills (ECPs), and they did not work. If she stays pregnant, will there be something wrong with her baby?

No. Studies have been done with women who did not know they were pregnant and kept taking birth control pills. These studies have found no greater risk for birth defects.

Is emergency contraception the same thing as the "abortion pill?"

No. Emergency contraception can keep a woman from becoming pregnant. It works one of the following three ways:

- By keeping the egg from leaving the ovary

- By keeping the sperm from meeting the egg

- By keeping the fertilized egg from attaching to the uterus (womb)

The abortion pill (Mifeprex, also called RU-486) works after a woman becomes pregnant (after a fertilized egg has attached to the uterus). The abortion pill makes the uterus force out the egg, ending the pregnancy.

Part Six

Sexually Transmitted Diseases

Chapter 60

Questions And Answers About Sexually Transmitted Diseases

What is a sexually transmitted disease (STD)?

It is an infection or disease passed from person to person through sexual contact.

How many people have STDs?

The United States has the highest rates of STDs in the industrialized world. In the United States alone, an estimated 15.3 million new cases of STDs are reported each year. Women suffer more frequent and more serious complications from STDs than men.

How do you get an STD?

You can get and pass STDs through vaginal, anal, or oral sex. Trichomoniasis can also be picked up from contact with damp or moist objects such as towels, wet clothing, or a toilet seat, if the genital area gets in contact with these damp objects. Some STDs cause no symptoms. But STDs can still be passed from person to person even if there are no symptoms.

About This Chapter: Information in this chapter is from "Sexually Transmitted Diseases: Overview," The National Women's Health Information Center, U.S. Department of Health and Human Services, Office on Women's Health, May 2005.

How do you get tested for STDs?

Talk with your doctor or nurse about getting tested for STDs. She or he can tell you how to test for each STD.

Can STDs cause health problems?

Yes. While each STD causes different health problems, overall, they can cause cervical cancer and other cancers, liver disease, pelvic inflammatory disease, infertility, pregnancy problems, and other complications. Some STDs

---

♣ **It's A Fact!!**

Heavy Drinking And Drug Use Linked To Higher Rates Of Sexually Transmitted Diseases Among Young Adults

Heavy drinking is linked to higher rates of sexually transmitted diseases among young adults, according to a report by the Substance Abuse and Mental Health Services Administration. Combined drug and alcohol use were associated with even higher STD rates.

Sexually Transmitted Diseases and Substance Use, based on data from the National Survey on Drug Use and Health 2005, showed that 3.1 percent of past month heavy drinkers ages 18 to 25 had an STD in the previous year, compared with 1.4 percent of young adults who did not drink in the past month. Heavy alcohol use involves consuming five or more drinks on the same occasion on five or more days in the past month.

When young adults used both illicit drugs and alcohol in the past month, the rate of reported STDs rose to 3.9 percent. Reported STDs in young adults were lowest for those who did not drink or use drugs during the past month (1.3 percent). Rates of reported STDs for those who used either an illicit drug or alcohol, but not both, were similar at 2.1 percent for both categories.

"Substance abuse and risky sexual behavior are closely connected," said Terry Cline, PhD, SAMHSA Administrator. "This report puts into sharp focus just one of the many potential lifetime consequences for young adults of heavy drinking and drug use. Unchecked heavy drinking and drug use can lead to serious dependence-related problems, including loss of friends and

increase your risk of getting human immunodeficiency virus/acquired immune deficiency syndrome (HIV/AIDS). HIV/AIDS can cause a number of health problems and raise the risk of getting life-threatening diseases and certain forms of cancer.

How are STDs treated?

The treatment depends on the type of STD. For some STDs, treatment may involve taking medicine or getting a shot. For other STDs that cannot be cured, like herpes, there is treatment to relieve the symptoms.

family, employment, housing, health, and even life. Young adults need to seriously consider the choices they are making and the impact those choices can have on their futures."

Overall, 0.8 percent of those 12 or older, about 2 million people, reported that they had been told by a doctor or other health professional that they had an STD in the past year. The rate was highest for 18 to 25 year olds (2.1 percent). Among adults, those 35 or older had the lowest rate of reported STDs at 0.5 percent.

Women had higher rates than men in all age groups, with women 18–25 being four times more likely than men in the same age group to have reported an STD. Other research shows that young women are more susceptible to certain STDs than are older women.

While both men's and women's STD rates rose with increasing alcohol use, the rate of reported STDs among female heavy drinkers reached 7.3 percent, compared with 1.3 percent of male heavy drinkers. A similar pattern of STD rates among young adults was found when illicit drug use and alcohol were combined. Women who used both alcohol and illicit drugs had a reported STD rate of 7.9 percent; for men who used both, the rate was 1.5 percent. Because studies show that women are more likely to be tested for STDs than men, comparing rates of diagnosed STDs may not provide the full picture of the difference in risk by gender.

Source: SAMHSA News Release, Substance Abuse and Mental Health Services Administration, March 2007.

What can I do to avoid getting an STD?

The following are steps you can take to keep from getting an STD:

- **Do not have sex.** The best way to prevent any STD is to practice abstinence, or not having vaginal, oral, or anal sex.

- **Be faithful.** Have a sexual relationship with one partner who has been tested for STDs and is not infected is another way to reduce your chances of getting infected. Be faithful to each other, meaning that you only have sex with each other and no one else.

- **Use condoms.** Protect yourself with a condom every time you have vaginal, anal, or oral sex. Condoms should be used for any type of sex with every partner. For vaginal sex, use a latex male condom or a female polyurethane condom. For anal sex, use a latex male condom. For oral sex, use a dental dam. A dental dam is a rubbery material that can be placed over the anus or the vagina before sexual contact.

- **Know that some methods of birth control, like birth control pills, shots, implants, or diaphragms, will not protect you from STDs.** If you use one of these methods, be sure to also use a latex condom or dental dam (used for oral sex) correctly every time you have sex.

- **Talk with your sex partner(s) about STDs and using condoms.** It is up to you to make sure you are protected. Remember, it is your body.

- **Talk frankly with your doctor or nurse and your sex partner(s) about any STDs you or your partner have or had.** Try not to be embarrassed.

- **Have regular pelvic exams.** Talk with your doctor about how often you need them. Many tests for STDs can be done during an exam. Ask your doctor to test you for STDs. The sooner an STD is found, the easier it is to treat.

Chapter 61

Chlamydia

What is chlamydia?

Chlamydia is a common sexually transmitted disease (STD) caused by the bacterium, *Chlamydia trachomatis*, which can damage a woman's reproductive organs. Even though symptoms of chlamydia are usually mild or absent, serious complications that cause irreversible damage, including infertility, can occur "silently" before a woman ever recognizes a problem. Chlamydia also can cause discharge from the penis of an infected man.

How common is chlamydia?

Chlamydia is the most frequently reported bacterial sexually transmitted disease in the United States. In 2004, 929,462 chlamydial infections were reported to the Centers for Disease Control and Prevention (CDC) from 50 states and the District of Columbia. Under reporting is substantial because most people with chlamydia are not aware of their infections and do not seek testing. Also, testing is not often done if patients are treated for their symptoms. An estimated 2.8 million Americans are infected with chlamydia each year. Women are frequently re-infected if their sex partners are not treated.

About This Chapter: Information in this chapter is from "Chlamydia—CDC Fact Sheet," Centers for Disease Control and Prevention, U.S. Department of Health and Human Services, April 2006.

How do people get chlamydia?

Chlamydia can be transmitted during vaginal, anal, or oral sex. Chlamydia can also be passed from an infected mother to her baby during vaginal childbirth.

Any sexually active person can be infected with chlamydia. The greater the number of sex partners, the greater the risk of infection. Since chlamydia can be transmitted by oral or anal sex, men who have sex with men are also at risk for chlamydial infection.

What are the symptoms of chlamydia?

Chlamydia is known as a "silent" disease because about three quarters of infected women and about half of infected men have no symptoms. If symptoms do occur, they usually appear within one to three weeks after exposure.

> ♣ **It's A Fact!!**
> Because the cervix (opening to the uterus) of teenage girls and young women is not fully matured, they are at particularly high risk for infection if sexually active.

In women, the bacteria initially infect the cervix and the urethra (urine canal). Women who have symptoms might have an abnormal vaginal discharge or a burning sensation when urinating. When the infection spreads from the cervix to the fallopian tubes (tubes that carry eggs from the ovaries to the uterus), some women still have no signs or symptoms; others have lower abdominal pain, low back pain, nausea, fever, pain during intercourse, or bleeding between menstrual periods. Chlamydial infection of the cervix can spread to the rectum.

Men with signs or symptoms might have a discharge from their penis or a burning sensation when urinating. Men might also have burning and itching around the opening of the penis. Pain and swelling in the testicles are uncommon.

Men or women who have receptive anal intercourse may acquire chlamydial infection in the rectum, which can cause rectal pain, discharge, or bleeding. Chlamydia can also be found in the throats of women and men having oral sex with an infected partner.

What complications can result from untreated chlamydia?

If untreated, chlamydial infections can progress to serious reproductive and other health problems with both short-term and long-term consequences. Like the disease itself, the damage that chlamydia causes is often "silent."

In women, untreated infection can spread into the uterus or fallopian tubes and cause pelvic inflammatory disease (PID). This happens in up to 40 percent of women with untreated chlamydia. PID can cause permanent damage to the fallopian tubes, uterus, and surrounding tissues. The damage can lead to chronic pelvic pain, infertility, and potentially fatal ectopic pregnancy (pregnancy outside the uterus). Women infected with chlamydia are up to five times more likely to become infected with human immunodeficiency virus (HIV), if exposed.

To help prevent the serious consequences of chlamydia, screening at least annually for chlamydia is recommended for all sexually active women age 25 years and younger. An annual screening test also is recommended for older women with risk factors for chlamydia (a new sex partner or multiple sex partners). All pregnant women should have a screening test for chlamydia.

Complications among men are rare. Infection sometimes spreads to the epididymis (a tube that carries sperm from the testis), causing pain, fever, and, rarely, sterility.

Rarely, genital chlamydial infection can cause arthritis that can be accompanied by skin lesions and inflammation of the eye and urethra (Reiter syndrome).

How is chlamydia diagnosed?

There are laboratory tests to diagnose chlamydia. Some can be performed on urine; other tests require that a specimen be collected from a site such as the penis or cervix.

What is the treatment for chlamydia?

Chlamydia can be easily treated and cured with antibiotics. A single dose of azithromycin or a week of doxycycline (twice daily) are the most commonly used treatments. HIV-positive persons with chlamydia should receive the same treatment as those who are HIV negative.

All sex partners should be evaluated, tested, and treated. Persons with chlamydia should abstain from sexual intercourse until they and their sex partners have completed treatment, otherwise re-infection is possible.

Women whose sex partners have not been appropriately treated are at high risk for re-infection. Having multiple infections increases a woman's risk of serious reproductive health complications, including infertility. Re-testing should be considered for women, especially adolescents, three to four months after treatment. This is especially true if a woman does not know if her sex partner received treatment.

How can chlamydia be prevented?

The surest way to avoid transmission of sexually transmitted diseases is to abstain from sexual contact, or to be in a long-term mutually monogamous relationship with a partner who has been tested and is known to be uninfected.

Latex male condoms, when used consistently and correctly, can reduce the risk of transmission of chlamydia.

Chlamydia screening is recommended annually for all sexually active women 25 years of age and younger. An annual screening test also is recommended for older women with risk factors for chlamydia (a new sex partner or multiple sex partners). All pregnant women should have a screening test for chlamydia.

Any genital symptoms, such as discharge or burning during urination or unusual sores or rash, should be a signal to stop having sex and to consult a health care provider immediately. If a person has been treated for chlamydia (or any other STD), he or she should notify all recent sex partners so they can see a health care provider and be treated. This will reduce the risk that the sex partners will develop serious complications from chlamydia and will also reduce the person's risk of becoming re-infected. The person and all of his or her sex partners must avoid sex until they have completed their treatment for chlamydia.

Chapter 62

Genital Herpes

What is genital herpes?

Genital herpes is a sexually transmitted disease caused by the herpes simplex viruses (HSV) type 1 and type 2. Most genital herpes is caused by HSV type 2.

Most people have no or minimal symptoms from HSV-1 or HSV-2 infection. When symptoms do occur, they usually appear as one or more blisters on or around the genitals or rectum. The blisters break, leaving ulcers or tender sores that may take up to four weeks to heal. Typically, another outbreak can appear weeks or months later.

Although the infection can stay in the body forever, the number of outbreaks usually decreases over a period of years. You can pass genital herpes to someone else even when you experience no symptoms.

How common is genital herpes?

About 45 million Americans, age 12 and older have genital herpes. It is estimated that up to one million people become infected each year. Genital herpes (HSV-2) is more common in women than men.

About This Chapter: The National Women's Health Information Center, U.S. Department of Health and Human Services, Office on Women's Health, May 2005.

How can I get genital herpes?

Herpes is a virus that can be passed through sexual contact. You can get genital herpes by having sex with someone who has open sores and when someone has no sores. However, herpes is most contagious when a person has open sores. People with herpes should not have sexual activity when sores or other symptoms of herpes are present. HSV-1 can cause genital herpes, but it more commonly causes infections of the mouth and lips or "fever blisters." Condoms can lower the chances of getting herpes. Along with condoms, Valtrex®, a drug used to treat herpes, can help lower the chances of passing the virus during vaginal sex.

What are the symptoms of genital herpes?

The symptoms of genital herpes vary from person to person. Some people have severe symptoms, such as many painful sores, while others have mild symptoms. An initial outbreak of genital herpes usually brings about symptoms within two weeks of having sexual contact with an infected person and can last from two to three weeks. The early symptoms can include the following:

- An itching or burning feeling in the genital or anal area

- Flu-like symptoms, including fever

- Swollen glands

- Pain in the legs, buttocks, or genital area

- Vaginal discharge

- A feeling of pressure in the area below the stomach

Within a few days, sores (also called lesions) show up where the virus has entered the body, such as on the mouth, penis, or vagina. Sores can also show up on a woman's cervix, which is the opening to the uterus or womb, or in the urinary passage in men. The sores are small red bumps that may turn into blisters or painful open sores. Over a period of days, the sores become crusted and then heal without scarring.

Other later symptoms of genital herpes may include the following:

- Small red bumps on the penis, vagina, or wherever the infection began. These bumps may become blisters or painful open sores that can take up to four weeks to heal.

- Itching or burning in the genital area

- Pain in the legs, buttocks, or genital area

- Vaginal discharge

- Feeling pressure or discomfort around your stomach

- Fever

- Headache

- Muscle aches

- Pain when urinating

- Swollen glands in the genital area

☞ Remember!!

If you have herpes, do not have any sexual activity with someone who does not have herpes when you have sores or other symptoms of herpes. Even if you do not have symptoms, you can still pass the virus to others.

Some people may have no symptoms, but they can still spread herpes. Sometimes only very mild sores appear but are mistaken for an insect bite or other skin problems. If you have human immunodeficiency virus (HIV), a genital herpes infection can be worse.

Can genital herpes come back?

Yes. Herpes symptoms can come and go, but the virus stays in the nerve cells of your body even after all signs of the infection have gone away. In most people, the virus becomes "active" from time to time, creating an outbreak. Some people have herpes virus outbreaks only once or twice. Other people have many outbreaks of herpes each year. Scientists do not know what causes the virus to become active, but the number of outbreaks a person has tends to go down over a period of years. Some women say the virus comes back when they are sick, under stress, out in the sun, or during their period.

How do I know for sure if I have genital herpes?

Doctors can diagnose genital herpes by looking at visible sores, if the outbreak is typical, and by taking a sample from the sore for testing in a lab.

Herpes can be difficult to diagnose between outbreaks. Blood tests, which detect HSV-1 or HSV-2 antibodies, can help to detect herpes in people without symptoms or during the time between outbreaks.

What is the treatment for genital herpes?

There is no treatment that can cure genital herpes; the virus will always be in your body. Certain drugs such as acyclovir, valacyclovir, and famciclovir can shorten outbreaks and make them less severe, or stop them from happening. Depending on your needs, your doctor can give you drugs to take right after getting outbreak symptoms or drugs that you can take on a regular basis to try to stop outbreaks from happening. When used along with safe sex practices, valacyclovir (brand name Valtrex®) can also help prevent you from passing the infection to someone else. Talk to your doctor about which treatment plan is best for you.

During outbreaks, these steps can speed healing and prevent spreading of the infection to other sites of the body or to other people:

- Keep the infected area clean and dry.

- Try not to touch the sores.

- Wash hands after contact.

- Avoid sexual contact from the time the symptoms are first noticed until the sores have healed.

> **♣ It's A Fact!!**
> Once you have the genital herpes, it stays in your body, and there is a chance that you will have outbreaks. Medicine can shorten and stop outbreaks from happening.

What can I do to prevent genital herpes?

These are things you can do to protect yourself from getting genital herpes:

- **Do not have sex.** The best way to prevent any sexually transmitted disease (STD) is to practice abstinence or not having vaginal, oral, or anal sex.

- **Be faithful.** Have a sexual relationship with one partner who has been tested for herpes, and is not infected, is another way to reduce your chances of getting infected. Be faithful to each other, meaning that you only have sex with each other and no one else.

- **Use condoms.** Protect yourself with a latex condom every time you have vaginal, anal, or oral sex. Condoms should be used for any type of sex with every partner. For vaginal sex, use a latex male condom or a female polyurethane condom. For anal sex, use a latex male condom. For oral sex, use a dental dam. A dental dam is a rubbery material that can be placed over the anus or the vagina before sexual contact.

- **Know that some methods of birth control, like birth control pills, shots, implants, or diaphragms, will not protect you from STDs.** If you use one of these methods, be sure to also use a latex condom or dental dam (used for oral sex) correctly every time you have sex.

- **Talk with your sex partner(s) about STDs and using latex condoms.** It is up to you to make sure you are protected.

- **Talk frankly with your doctor or nurse and your sex partner(s) about any STDs you or your partner have or had.** Try not to be embarrassed.

- **Know the symptoms.** Learn the common symptoms of genital herpes and other STDs. Seek medical help right away if you think you may have genital herpes or another STD.

What should I do if I have genital herpes?

- See your doctor for testing and treatment right away.

- Follow your doctor's orders and finish all the medicine that you are given. Even if the symptoms go away, you still need to finish all of the medicine.

- Avoid having any sexual activity while you are being treated for genital herpes and while you have any symptoms of an outbreak.

- Be sure to tell your sexual partners, so they can be tested.

- Remember that genital herpes is a life long disease. Even though you may have long periods with no symptoms, you can still pass the virus to another person. Talk with your doctor about what you can do to have fewer future outbreaks and how to prevent passing the virus to another person.

Chapter 63

Gonorrhea

What is gonorrhea?

Gonorrhea is a sexually transmitted disease (STD). Gonorrhea is caused by *Neisseria gonorrhoeae*, a bacterium that can grow and multiply easily in the warm, moist areas of the reproductive tract, including the cervix (opening to the womb), uterus (womb), and fallopian tubes (egg canals) in women, and in the urethra (urine canal) in women and men. The bacterium can also grow in the mouth, throat, eyes, and anus.

How common is gonorrhea?

Gonorrhea is a very common infectious disease. Centers for Disease Control and Prevention (CDC) estimates that more than 700,000 persons in the United States get new gonorrheal infections each year. Only about half of these infections are reported to CDC. In 2004, 330,132 cases of gonorrhea were reported to CDC. In the period from 1975 to 1997, the national gonorrhea rate declined, following the implementation of the national gonorrhea control program in the mid-1970s. After a small increase in 1998, the gonorrhea rate has decreased slightly since 1999. In 2004, the rate of reported gonorrheal infections was 113.5 per 100,000 persons.

About This Chapter: Centers for Disease Control and Prevention, U.S. Department of Health and Human Services, April 2006.

How do people get gonorrhea?

Gonorrhea is spread through contact with the penis, vagina, mouth, or anus. Ejaculation does not have to occur for gonorrhea to be transmitted or acquired. Gonorrhea can also be spread from mother to baby during delivery.

People who have had gonorrhea and received treatment may get infected again if they have sexual contact with a person infected with gonorrhea.

What are the signs and symptoms of gonorrhea?

Although many men with gonorrhea may have no symptoms at all, some men have some signs or symptoms that appear two to five days after infection; symptoms can take as long as 30 days to appear. Symptoms and signs include a burning sensation when urinating, or a white, yellow, or green discharge from the penis. Sometimes men with gonorrhea get painful or swollen testicles.

♣ **It's A Fact!!**
Who Is At Risk For Gonorrhea?

Any sexually active person can be infected with gonorrhea. In the United States, the highest reported rates of infection are among sexually active teenagers, young adults, and African Americans.

In women, the symptoms of gonorrhea are often mild, but most women who are infected have no symptoms. Even when a woman has symptoms, they can be so non-specific as to be mistaken for a bladder or vaginal infection. The initial symptoms and signs in women include a painful or burning sensation when urinating, increased vaginal discharge, or vaginal bleeding between periods. Women with gonorrhea are at risk of developing serious complications from the infection, regardless of the presence or severity of symptoms.

Symptoms of rectal infection in both men and women may include discharge, anal itching, soreness, bleeding, or painful bowel movements. Rectal infection also may cause no symptoms. Infections in the throat may cause a sore throat but usually causes no symptoms.

What are the complications of gonorrhea?

Untreated gonorrhea can cause serious and permanent health problems in both women and men.

In women, gonorrhea is a common cause of pelvic inflammatory disease (PID). About one million women each year in the United States develop PID. Women with PID do not necessarily have symptoms. When symptoms are present, they can be very severe and can include abdominal pain and fever. PID can lead to internal abscesses (pus-filled "pockets" that are hard to cure) and long-lasting, chronic pelvic pain. PID can damage the fallopian tubes enough to cause infertility or increase the risk of ectopic pregnancy. Ectopic pregnancy is a life-threatening condition in which a fertilized egg grows outside the uterus, usually in a fallopian tube.

In men, gonorrhea can cause epididymitis, a painful condition of the testicles that can lead to infertility if left untreated.

Gonorrhea can spread to the blood or joints. This condition can be life threatening. In addition, people with gonorrhea can more easily contract human immunodeficiency virus (HIV), the virus that causes acquired immune deficiency syndrome (AIDS). HIV-infected people with gonorrhea are more likely to transmit HIV to someone else.

How is gonorrhea diagnosed?

Several laboratory tests are available to diagnose gonorrhea. A doctor or nurse can obtain a sample for testing from the parts of the body likely to be infected (cervix, urethra, rectum, or throat) and send the sample to a laboratory for analysis. Gonorrhea that is present in the cervix or urethra can be diagnosed in a laboratory by testing a urine sample. A quick laboratory test for gonorrhea that can be done in some clinics or doctor's offices is a Gram stain. A Gram stain of a sample from a urethra or a cervix allows the doctor to see the gonorrhea bacterium under a microscope. This test works better for men than for women.

What is the treatment for gonorrhea?

Several antibiotics can successfully cure gonorrhea in adolescents and adults. However, drug-resistant strains of gonorrhea are increasing in many areas of the world, including the United States, and successful treatment of gonorrhea is becoming more difficult. Because many people with gonorrhea also have chlamydia, another sexually transmitted disease, antibiotics for both infections are usually given together. Persons with gonorrhea should be tested for other STDs.

It is important to take all of the medication prescribed to cure gonorrhea. Although medication will stop the infection, it will not repair any permanent damage done by the disease. People who have had gonorrhea and have been treated can get the disease again if they have sexual contact with persons infected with gonorrhea. If a person's symptoms continue even after receiving treatment, he or she should return to a doctor to be reevaluated.

How can gonorrhea be prevented?

The surest way to avoid transmission of sexually transmitted diseases is to abstain from sexual intercourse, or to be in a long-term mutually monogamous relationship with a partner who has been tested and is known to be uninfected.

Latex condoms, when used consistently and correctly, can reduce the risk of transmission of gonorrhea.

Any genital symptoms such as discharge or burning during urination or unusual sores or rash should be a signal to stop having sex and to see a doctor immediately. If a person has been diagnosed and treated for gonorrhea, he or she should notify all recent sex partners so they can see a health care provider and be treated. This will reduce the risk that the sex partners will develop serious complications from gonorrhea and will also reduce the person's risk of becoming re-infected. The person and all of his or her sex partners must avoid sex until they have completed their treatment for gonorrhea.

Chapter 64

Hepatitis B

What is hepatitis?

Hepatitis means inflammation (or swelling) of the liver.

If a virus causes the inflammation, it is called viral hepatitis. Different hepatitis viruses have been given different names, such as A, B, and C. A hepatitis virus is one that lives in liver cells.

When the liver is inflamed, it can have a harder time doing some of its jobs.

What is hepatitis B?

Hepatitis B is a disease that affects your liver. The hepatitis B virus causes it. Most people who get hepatitis B can get rid of the virus on their own, but others can develop chronic (or lifelong) hepatitis B.

Who is at risk of hepatitis B?

The Centers for Disease Control and Prevention (CDC) say that these groups are more likely to get hepatitis B:

- Persons with multiple sex partners or diagnosis of a sexually transmitted disease

- Men who have sex with men

About This Chapter: Information in this chapter is from "Basics," National Hepatitis C Program, United States Department of Veterans Affairs, February 2007.

- Sex contacts of infected persons

- Injection drug users

- Household contacts of chronically infected persons

- Infants born to infected mothers

- Infants and children of immigrants from areas with high rates of hepatitis B, particularly Africa, Asia, Alaska, and parts of South America

- Health care and public safety workers

- Hemodialysis patients (or people who use a kidney machine)

> ✔ **Quick Tip**
> **How To Protect Yourself Against Hepatitis B**
>
> - Practice safer sex. Use condoms every time you have sex.
>
> - Do not shoot drugs. If you are using drugs now, try to get help to stop. If you cannot stop, then do not share needles and works.
>
> - Do not share personal care items like razors, toothbrushes, and nail clippers.

How can you protect yourself against hepatitis B?

Get Vaccinated: There is a vaccine that protects you from getting hepatitis B. You get it in three different shots. Most people who get these shots develop antibodies. Antibodies are proteins that your body makes to fight certain diseases. These antibodies will protect you against hepatitis B. If you already got vaccinated, or if you are not sure, talk with your doctor (or health care provider). Your health care provider can check to see if you have antibodies against hepatitis B.

Avoid High-Risk Behaviors: High-risk behaviors are things that some people do that make them more likely to get a disease. You can get hepatitis B through contact with (or by touching) the blood of a person who has the disease. You can also get hepatitis B through contact with other body fluids like semen and vaginal fluids. For example, you can get hepatitis B by having sex or sharing needles with a person who has the disease.

If you can stop high-risk behaviors like these, it can also prevent you from getting other viruses like human immunodeficiency virus (HIV) and hepatitis C virus. Please speak with your doctor or nurse to get more information about these viruses.

Will you know if you have hepatitis B?

Not necessarily. You may have hepatitis B and not have any symptoms. You can still spread the virus to others even if you do not have symptoms. Some people who do have symptoms might have the following:

- Yellowing skin or eyes (or jaundice)

- Not feeling hungry

- Feeling tired

- Muscle, joint, or stomach pain

- Stomach upset, diarrhea, or vomiting

What are the tests for hepatitis B?

Your doctor may ask you to do the following tests:

- **Hepatitis B surface antibody (*Anti-HBs*):** If this test is positive, it means that you have antibodies against hepatitis B and are safe from getting the disease, and you were either vaccinated against hepatitis B or exposed to it at some point in your lifetime.

- **Hepatitis B core antibody (*Anti-HBc*):** If the test is positive, it means that you have been exposed to hepatitis B and have developed an antibody to only part of the virus, and they will do more tests to find out if you have the disease.

- **Hepatitis B surface antigen (*HBsAg*):** If this test is positive, it means that you do have hepatitis B, and you can spread the virus to others.

- **Hepatitis B e antigen (*HBeAg*):** If this test is positive, it means that you have high levels of virus in your blood, and you may be very contagious to others.

Is hepatitis B serious?

Yes. Although many people who are exposed to hepatitis B will be able to get rid of the virus, some people can develop chronic (or lifelong) hepatitis B. This may lead to liver damage, liver cancer, and death.

Are there treatments for hepatitis B?

There are five Food and Drug Administration (FDA)-approved drugs for the treatment of hepatitis B: interferon, pegylated interferon, lamivudine, entecavir, and adefovir. Your doctor can determine if medicine is needed for you and which medication to use.

What is the hepatitis B vaccine?

A vaccine is a shot of inactive virus that stimulates your natural immune system. After you get the hepatitis B vaccine, your body will make antibodies that will protect you against the virus. These antibodies are stored in your body for several years and will fight off the hepatitis B virus if you are exposed to it.

Who should get the hepatitis B vaccine?

You may need the hepatitis B vaccine if you:

- have a chronic liver disease, such as hepatitis C;

- live in, or were born in, areas where hepatitis B is common;

- inject drugs;

- have a sex partner who has hepatitis B or have multiple sex partners;

- are a man who has sex with other men;

- share a household with someone who has hepatitis B;

- work in a high-risk profession, especially if you are a health care worker, emergency worker, police officer, firefighter, mortician, or work in the military;

- are an international traveler;

- are in prison;

- receive blood products or are on hemodialysis.

> ♣ **It's A Fact!!**
> Certain ethnic groups have higher rates of hepatitis B virus infection. You may need the vaccine if you are African-American, Latino, Native American, Haitian, Alaskan Native, Vietnamese, Chinese, Korean, or Filipino.

How is the hepatitis B vaccine given?

For both children and adults, the vaccine should be given as three shots. The vaccine is given as follows: a single shot, followed by a second injection one month later, and then a third shot six months later. People who are infected with another virus, such as the human immunodeficiency virus (HIV), or who have problems with their immune system, may need larger doses of the hepatitis B vaccine.

Babies born to infected mothers should get the first shot within 12 hours after birth, followed by a second shot one month later, and the third shot six months later. Babies born to mothers who are not infected with the hepatitis B virus should get the first shot within one to two months after birth, and the second shot a month later, and the third shot six months later.

You will not get hepatitis B from the vaccine.

What if you do not get hepatitis B shots on time?

If you are not able to get the shots on time, the vaccine may still work if you get your second and third shots at least two months apart from each other. Ask your doctor for more information.

How long will the hepatitis B vaccine protect you?

You will be protected for about 13 years. If it has been many years since you received your hepatitis B vaccine, or if you do not know when you were vaccinated, ask your doctor to check to see if you have antibodies against hepatitis B.

What should you do if you are exposed to the hepatitis B virus?

If you know you were recently exposed to the hepatitis B virus, you may get protection from a shot of hepatitis B immunoglobulin (HBIG) within 24 hours after your exposure. This will protect you for three to six months, but it is also strongly recommended that you begin the three-shot hepatitis B vaccine series, starting within seven days of your exposure.

What are the side effects of the hepatitis B vaccine?

There are very few side effects, the most common being soreness where you got the shot. You will not get hepatitis B from the vaccine. Pregnant women have received the hepatitis B vaccine with no risk to the baby.

Chapter 65

Human Immunodeficiency Virus (HIV) And Acquired Immune Deficiency Syndrome (AIDS)

Overview

AIDS was first reported in the United States in 1981 and has since become a major worldwide epidemic. The human immunodeficiency virus, or HIV, causes AIDS. By killing or damaging cells of the body's immune system, HIV progressively destroys the body's ability to fight infections and certain cancers. People diagnosed with AIDS may get life-threatening diseases called opportunistic infections. These infections are caused by microbes such as viruses or bacteria that usually do not make healthy people sick.

Transmission

HIV is spread most often through unprotected sex with an infected partner. The virus can enter the body through the lining of the vagina, vulva, penis, rectum, or mouth during sex.

About This Chapter: Information in this chapter is excerpted from "HIV Infection and AIDS: An Overview," National Institute of Allergy and Infectious Diseases, National Institutes of Health, U.S. Department of Health and Human Services, October 2007.

Risky Behavior

HIV can infect anyone who practices risky behaviors such as sharing drug needles or syringes; having sexual contact, including oral sexual contact, with an infected person without using a condom; having sexual contact with someone whose HIV status is unknown.

♣ It's A Fact!!
Since 1981, more than 980,000 cases of AIDS have been reported in the United States to the Centers for Disease Control and Prevention (CDC). According to CDC, more than 1,000,000 Americans may be infected with HIV, one-quarter of whom are unaware of their infection.

Infected Blood

HIV also is spread through contact with infected blood. Before donated blood was screened for evidence of HIV infection and before heat-treating techniques to destroy HIV in blood products were introduced, HIV was transmitted through transfusions of contaminated blood or blood components. Today, because of blood screening and heat treatment, the risk of getting HIV from blood transfusions is extremely small.

Contaminated Needles

HIV is often spread among injection drug users when they share needles or syringes contaminated with very small quantities of blood from someone infected with the virus.

It is rare for a patient to be the source of HIV transmitted to a healthcare provider or vice versa by accidental sticks with contaminated needles or other medical instruments.

Saliva

Although researchers have found HIV in the saliva of infected people, there is no evidence that the virus is spread by contact with saliva. Laboratory studies reveal that saliva has natural properties that limit the power of HIV to infect, and the amount of virus in saliva appears to be very low. Research studies of people infected with HIV have found no evidence that the virus is spread to others through saliva by kissing. HIV, however, can infect the lining of the mouth, and instances of HIV transmission through oral intercourse have been reported.

Scientists have found no evidence that HIV is spread through sweat, tears, urine, or feces.

Sexually Transmitted Infections

People with a sexually transmitted infection, such as syphilis, genital herpes, chlamydia, gonorrhea, or bacterial vaginosis, may be more susceptible to getting HIV infection during sex with infected partners.

Symptoms

Early Symptoms

Many people will not have any symptoms when they first become infected with HIV. They may, however, have a flu-like illness within a month or two after exposure to the virus. This illness may include fever, headache, tiredness, and enlarged lymph nodes (glands of the immune system easily felt in the neck and groin).

These symptoms usually disappear within a week to a month and are often mistaken for those of another viral infection. During this period, people are very infectious, and HIV is present in large quantities in genital fluids.

♣ **It's A Fact!!**
Studies of families of HIV-infected people have shown clearly that HIV is not spread through casual contact such as the sharing of food utensils, towels and bedding, swimming pools, telephones, or toilet seats.

HIV is not spread by biting insects such as mosquitoes or bedbugs.

Later Symptoms

More persistent or severe symptoms may not appear for ten years or more after HIV first enters the body in adults, or within two years in children born with HIV infection. This period of asymptomatic infection varies greatly in each person. Some people may begin to have symptoms within a few months, while others may be symptom-free for more than ten years.

Even during the asymptomatic period, the virus is actively multiplying, infecting, and killing cells of the immune system. The virus can also hide within infected cells and be inactive. The most obvious effect of HIV infection is a decline in the number of CD4 positive T (CD4+) cells found in the blood—the immune system's key infection fighters. The virus slowly disables or destroys these cells without causing symptoms.

As the immune system becomes more debilitated, a variety of complications start to take over. For many people, the first signs of infection are large lymph nodes, or swollen glands that may be enlarged for more than three months. Other symptoms often experienced months to years before the onset of AIDS include lack of energy; weight loss; frequent fevers and sweats; persistent or frequent yeast infections (oral or vaginal); persistent skin rashes or flaky skin; pelvic inflammatory disease in women that does not respond to treatment; short-term memory loss.

Some people develop frequent and severe herpes infections that cause mouth, genital, or anal sores, or a painful nerve disease called shingles. Children may grow slowly or get sick frequently.

What Is AIDS?

Symptoms of opportunistic infections common in people with AIDS include the following:

- Coughing and shortness of breath

- Seizures and lack of coordination

- Difficult or painful swallowing

- Mental symptoms such as confusion and forgetfulness

- Severe and persistent diarrhea

- Fever

- Vision loss

- Nausea, abdominal cramps, and vomiting

- Weight loss and extreme fatigue

- Severe headaches

- Coma

Children with AIDS may get the same opportunistic infections, as do adults with the disease. In addition, they also may have severe forms of the typically common childhood bacterial infections, such as conjunctivitis (pink eye), ear infections, and tonsillitis.

People with AIDS are also particularly prone to developing various cancers, especially those caused by viruses such as Kaposi sarcoma and cervical cancer, or cancers of the immune system known as lymphomas. These cancers are usually more aggressive and difficult to treat in people with AIDS. Signs of Kaposi sarcoma in light-skinned people are round brown, reddish, or purple spots that develop in the skin or in the mouth. In dark-skinned people, the spots are more pigmented.

Diagnosis

Because early HIV infection often causes no symptoms, a healthcare provider usually can diagnose it by testing blood for the presence of antibodies (disease-fighting proteins) to HIV. HIV antibodies generally do not reach noticeable levels in the blood for one to three months after infection. It may take the antibodies as long as six months to be produced in quantities large enough to show up in standard blood tests. Hence, to determine whether a person has been recently infected (acute infection), a healthcare provider can screen blood for the presence of HIV genetic material. Direct screening of HIV is extremely critical in order to prevent transmission of HIV from recently infected individuals.

Anyone who has been exposed to the virus should get an HIV test as soon as the immune system is likely to develop antibodies to the virus—within 6 weeks to 12 months after possible exposure to the virus. By getting tested early, a healthcare provider can give advice to an infected person about when to start treatment to help the immune system combat HIV and help prevent the emergence of certain opportunistic infections. Early testing also alerts an infected person to avoid high-risk behaviors that could spread the virus to others.

Most healthcare providers can do HIV testing and will usually offer counseling at the same time. Of course, testing can be done anonymously at many sites if a person is concerned about confidentiality.

Treatment

HIV Infection

The Food and Drug Administration (FDA) has approved a number of drugs for treating HIV infection. The first group of drugs, called reverse transcriptase (RT) inhibitors, interrupts an early stage of the virus making copies of itself. Nucleoside/nucleotide RT inhibitors are faulty DNA building blocks. When these faulty pieces are incorporated into the HIV DNA (during the process when the HIV RNA is converted to HIV DNA), the DNA chain cannot be completed, thereby blocking HIV from replicating in a cell. Non-nucleoside RT inhibitors bind to reverse transcriptase, interfering with its ability to convert the HIV RNA into HIV DNA. This class of drugs may slow the spread of HIV in the body and delay the start of opportunistic infections.

FDA has approved a second class of drugs for treating HIV infection. These drugs, called protease inhibitors, interrupt the virus from making copies of itself at a later step in its life cycle.

FDA also has introduced a third new class of drugs, known at fusion inhibitors, to treat HIV infection. Fuzeon (enfuvirtide or T-20), the first approved fusion inhibitor, works by interfering with the ability of HIV-1 to enter into cells by blocking the merging of the virus with the cell membranes. This inhibition blocks HIV's ability to enter and infect the human immune cells. Fuzeon is designed for use in combination with other anti-HIV treatments. It reduces the level of HIV infection in the blood and may be effective against HIV that has become resistant to current antiviral treatment schedules.

Opportunistic Infections

A number of available drugs help treat opportunistic infections such as eye infections, yeast and other fungal infections, and PCP (*Pneumocystis carinii* pneumonia).

Cancers

Healthcare providers use radiation, chemotherapy, or injections of alpha interferon, a genetically engineered protein that occurs naturally in the human body, to treat Kaposi sarcoma or other cancers associated with HIV infection.

Prevention

Many people infected with HIV have no symptoms. Therefore, there is no way of knowing with certainty whether a sexual partner is infected unless he or she has repeatedly tested negative for the virus and has not engaged in any risky behavior. Abstaining from having sex or using male latex condoms or female polyurethane condoms may offer partial protection during oral, anal, or vaginal sex. Only water-based lubricants should be used with male latex condoms.

Although some laboratory evidence shows that spermicides can kill HIV, researchers have not found that these products can prevent a person from getting HIV.

♣ It's A Fact!!

Because there is no vaccine for HIV, the only way people can prevent infection with the virus is to avoid behaviors putting them at risk of infection, such as sharing needles and having unprotected sex.

Chapter 66

Human Papillomavirus

What Is Human Papillomavirus (HPV)?

Human papillomavirus (HPV) is a sexually transmitted virus. It is passed on through genital contact (such as vaginal and anal sex). It is also passed on by skin-to-skin contact. At least 50% of people who have had sex will have HPV at some time in their lives.

Why haven't I heard of HPV?

HPV is not a new virus, but many people do not know about it. Most people do not have any signs. HPV may go away on its own without causing any health problems.

Who can get HPV?

Anyone who has ever had genital contact with another person may have HPV. Both men and women may get it, and pass it on without knowing it. Since there might not be any signs, a person may have HPV even if years have passed since he or she had sex.

About This Chapter: Information under the heading "What Is Human Papillomavirus (HPV)?" is from "HPV (human papillomavirus)," U.S. Food and Drug Administration, Office of Women's Health, U.S. Department of Health and Human Services, June 2006. Text under the heading "Cervical Cancer Vaccine," is excerpted from "Cervical Cancer Vaccine Continues to Spark Debate," National Women's Health Information Center, U.S. Department of Health and Human Services, March 2007.

What makes a person more likely to get HPV?

Most people who have sex may get HPV. You are more likely to get HPV if you have:

- sex at an early age,

- many sex partners, or

- a sex partner who has had many partners.

If there are no signs, why do I need to worry about HPV?

There are many kinds of HPV and not all of them cause health problems. Some kinds of HPV may cause problems like genital warts or cervical cancer. HPV types 16 and 18 cause about 70% of cervical cancers. HPV types 6 and 11 cause about 90% of genital warts.

Is there a cure for HPV?

There is no cure for the virus (HPV) itself. There are treatments for the health problems that HPV can cause, such as genital warts, cervical changes, and cervical cancer.

What should I know about genital warts?

There are many treatment choices for genital warts; but even after the warts are treated, the virus might still be there and may be passed on to others. If genital warts are not treated they may go away, stay the same, or increase in size or number, but they will not turn into cancer.

What should I know about cervical cancer?

All women should get regular Pap tests. The Pap test looks for cell changes caused by HPV. The test finds cell changes early so the cervix can be treated before the cells turn into cancer. This test also can also find cancer in its early stages so it can be treated before it becomes too serious. It is rare to die from cervical cancer if the disease is caught early.

Is there a test for HPV?

Yes. It tests for the kinds of HPV that may lead to cervical cancer. The U.S. Food and Drug Administration (FDA) approved the HPV test to be used for

✤ It's A Fact!!
Risk Factors For Cervical Cancer

Doctors cannot always explain why one woman develops cervical cancer and another does not. However, we do know that a woman with certain risk factors may be more likely than others to develop cervical cancer.

Studies have found a number of factors that may increase the risk of cervical cancer. These factors may act together to increase the risk even more:

- **Human papillomaviruses (HPVs):** HPV infection is the main risk factor for cervical cancer.

- **Lack of regular Pap tests:** Cervical cancer is more common among women who do not have regular Pap tests. The Pap test helps doctors find precancerous cells. Treating precancerous cervical changes often prevents cancer.

- **Weakened immune system (the body's natural defense system):** Women with human immunodeficiency virus (HIV) infection or who take drugs that suppress the immune system have a higher-than-average risk of developing cervical cancer.

- **Age:** Cancer of the cervix occurs most often in women over the age of 40.

- **Sexual history:** Women who have had many sexual partners have a higher-than-average risk of developing cervical cancer. Also, a woman who has had sexual intercourse with a man who has had many sexual partners may be at higher risk of developing cervical cancer.

- **Smoking cigarettes:** Women with an HPV infection who smoke cigarettes have a higher risk of cervical cancer than women with HPV infection who do not smoke.

- **Using birth control pills for a long time:** Using birth control pills for a long time (five or more years) may increase the risk of cervical cancer among women with HPV infection.

- **Having many children:** Studies suggest that giving birth to many children may increase the risk of cervical cancer among women with HPV infection.

Women who think they may be at risk for cancer of the cervix should discuss this concern with their doctor. They may want to ask about a schedule for checkups.

Source: Excerpted from "Risk Factors," What You Need To Know About™ Cancer of the Cervix, National Cancer Institute, U.S. National Institutes of Health, March 2005.

women over 30 years old. It may find HPV even before there are changes to the cervix. Women who have the HPV test still need to get the Pap test.

Can I lower my chances of getting HPV?

- You can choose not to have sex (abstinence).

- If you have sex, you can limit the number of partners you have.

- Choose a partner who has had no or few sex partners. The fewer partners your partner has had, the less likely he or she is to have HPV.

- It is not known how much condoms protect against HPV. Areas not covered by a condom can be exposed to the virus.

What is the HPV vaccine and how does it work?

The vaccine, called Gardasil, mimics the disease and creates resistance. It is not a live or a dead virus. It prevents infection with HPV types 6, 11, 16, and 18.

Is it safe?

Tests of the vaccine showed only minor problems. Some people had a slight fever. Others had redness or irritation on their skin where they got the shot.

Is it effective?

Gardasil is between 95–100% effective against HPV types 6, 11, 16, and 18.

Who should get the HPV vaccine?

The FDA has approved Gardasil for girls and women ages 9–26. It is best to get the shot before the start of sexual activity.

How many shots do you need?

There are three shots. Once you get the first shot, you need a second shot two months later. You need to get a third shot six months after you get the first shot.

How long are you protected?

Since the vaccine is new, more studies need to be done. For example, the FDA does not know if you will need to have a booster after a couple of years.

Should I get the vaccine if I already have HPV?

The vaccine will not treat or cure HPV. It may help people who have one type of HPV from being infected with the other types. For example, if you have type 6, it may protect you from getting type 16.

Can I catch HPV from getting the vaccine?

No. The vaccine does not contain the HPV virus.

Cervical Cancer Vaccine

As states consider laws that would require girls entering sixth grade to be vaccinated against the cervical cancer-causing HPV, the morality behind the move has taken center stage.

Some experts support mandating vaccination for all girls, while others support voluntary use of the vaccine. Conservative groups and some parents have also voiced the concern that immunizing girls against HPV, which is transmitted sexually, might lead to more premarital sex.

Routine, voluntary use of the vaccine in young girls does have the support of most major U.S. medical groups. In fact, the U.S. Centers for Disease Control and Prevention's Advisory Committee on Immunization Practice formally recommended use of the vaccine for girls aged 11 and 12, and for females aged 13 to 26 who have not yet been immunized.

"The vaccine is an important vaccine, and it has the ability to decrease cancer," said Dr. Robert Frenck, a professor of pediatrics at Cincinnati Children's Hospital. "My concern is that HPV is a different kind of transmission than diseases we normally look at for mandating vaccines," Frenck said. "Diseases such as measles or chickenpox are transmitted by casual contact. With HPV, it's not a casual contact."

In addition, Frenck believes there will be significant economic consequences for states if the HPV vaccine is mandated. Pending bills that mandate the vaccine have provisions for the state to pay for immunization, he noted. That could turn out to be very expensive.

"Right now, the three-dose series is approximately $120 a dose—that's $360 for the full series," he said. Without extra funds, the cost of the vaccine would strain already overburdened public health systems, he said.

Another expert is also against mandating the vaccine, but this time for medical reasons.

"The vaccine is too new to be thinking about mandates," said Dr. Jon Abramson, a professor of infectious diseases at Wake Forest University Medical School and chairman of the CDC's immunization practices committee.

His committee does not consider recommending mandating a vaccine until it has been available for a long period of time, so that they can properly judge the demand, Abramson said. "We never discussed mandates, because it was way too early," he noted.

Because HPV is sexually transmitted, it also does not present the same risk as diseases that are transmitted by more casual contact, he added. "Most of the things we have mandates for are things that are high-risk in a school setting," Abramson said. "If someone walks into a school with measles, it's going to rapidly spread to those who aren't protected. Hopefully, you are at lower risk for HPV in school."

Finally, most state-proposed mandates include an easy way for parents to waive the HPV vaccine requirement. That worries Abramson, because it might make it easier for parents to opt out of other mandated vaccines, as well. "That will harm our other vaccines," he said.

To those who think that money is an issue in mandating the vaccine, Dr. Ralph Anderson, chairman of obstetrics and gynecology at the University of North Texas Health Center, said they need to prove that it costs more to vaccinate girls than to treat them for cervical cancer later in life.

♣ **It's A Fact!!**
Despite some public opposition to mandates, many medical professionals feel strongly that the vaccine should be mandated, because it can prevent up to 70 percent of cervical cancers.

Source: National Women's Health Information Center

"It costs $300 to get the vaccine. If you get cancer of the cervix, it will probably cost $100,000 to treat it, and then a lot of those people die," he said. "Show me that it's more expensive to give the vaccine than not give the vaccine. The cost concern is a smokescreen."

Not all the objections to mandating the vaccine are medical. Others have voiced political and moral objections.

"It's an end run around parental rights," said Wendy Wright, president of Concerned Women for America, a conservative lobbying group. "Parents know what's best for their daughters. Even with an opt-out option, it puts the parents in a position where they have to justify themselves to government officials," she said.

Chapter 67

Molluscum Contagiosum

Molluscum contagiosum is a common skin disease that is caused by a virus. The disease is generally mild and should not be a reason for concern or worry.

Molluscum infection causes small white, pink, or flesh-colored bumps or growths with a dimple or pit in the center. The bumps are usually smooth and firm and can appear anywhere on the body. They may become sore, red, and swollen but are usually painless. The bumps normally disappear within 6 to 12 months without treatment and without leaving scars. In people with weakened immune systems, molluscum growths may grow very large, spread more easily to other parts of the body, and may be harder to cure.

How It Spreads

People with this skin disease can cause the bumps to spread to different parts of their body. This is called autoinoculation. Such spread can occur by touching or scratching a bump and then touching another part of the body.

The virus can also be spread from person to person. This can happen if the growths on one person are touched by another person. It can also happen if the virus gets on an object that is touched by other people. Examples of such objects are towels, clothing, and toys. Molluscum can also be spread

About This Chapter: Information in this chapter is from "An Overview of Molluscum Contagiosum," Centers for Disease Control and Prevention, U.S. Department of Health and Human Services, August 2006.

from one person to another by sexual contact. Anyone who develops bumps in the genital area (on or near the penis, vulva, vagina, or anus) should see a health care provider. Bumps in these areas sometimes mean that molluscum or some other disease was spread through sexual contact.

How To Prevent The Spread Of Molluscum

Wash Your Hands

There are ways to prevent the spread of molluscum contagiosum. The best way is to follow good hygiene (cleanliness) habits. Keeping your hands clean is the best way to avoid molluscum infection, as well as many other infections. Hand washing removes germs that may have been picked up from other people or from surfaces that have germs on them.

Don't Scratch Or Pick At Molluscum Bumps

It is important not to touch, pick, or scratch skin that has bumps or blisters—that includes not only your own skin but also anyone else's. Picking and scratching can spread the virus to other parts of the body and makes it easier to spread the disease to other people too.

Keep Molluscum Bumps Covered

It is important to keep the area with molluscum growths clean and covered with clothing or a bandage so that others do not touch the bumps and become infected with molluscum. Do remember to keep the affected skin clean and dry.

However, when there is no risk of others coming into contact with your skin, such as at night when you sleep, uncover the bumps to help keep your skin healthy.

Sports And Activities To Avoid Or Be Careful With When You Have Molluscum

To prevent spread of the infection to other people, people with molluscum should not take part in contact sports unless clothing or bandages can cover all growths. Wrestling, basketball, and football are examples of contact sports.

Activities that use shared gear should also be avoided unless all bumps can be covered. Helmets, baseball gloves, and balls are examples of shared gear.

Swimming should also be avoided unless watertight bandages can cover all growths. Personal items (such as towels, goggles, and swim suits) should not be shared. Other items and equipment (such as kick boards and water toys) should be used only when clothing or watertight bandages cover all bumps.

Other Ways To Avoid Sharing Your Infection

- People with molluscum should not share other personal items that may spread the virus. Some examples of personal items are unwashed clothes, hairbrushes, wristwatches, and bar soap.

- People with molluscum should not shave or have electrolysis performed on body areas that have growths.

- People who have bumps in the genital area (on or near the penis, vulva, vagina, or anus) should avoid sexual contact until they have seen a health care provider.

Treating Molluscum

Some treatments exist for molluscum that may prevent spread of the infection to other parts of the body and to other people. A health care provider can remove the growths with surgery or laser therapy. A health care provider may also prescribe a cream to apply on the bumps or a medicine to take by mouth.

> **✔ Quick Tip**
>
> Some molluscum treatments that are advertised on the internet are not effective and may even be harmful. Therefore, always discuss any therapy with a health care provider before using it.

However, treatment is not usually required because the bumps disappear on their own within six months. However, they may not go away completely for up to four years. In addition, not all treatments are successful for all people. For example, it is more difficult to treat persons who have a weak immune system. This includes people who are infected with human immunodeficiency virus (HIV) or who are receiving drugs to treat cancer.

Chapter 68

Nongonococcal Urethritis

What Is Nongonococcal Urethritis (NGU)?

Nongonococcal urethritis is an infection of the urethra caused by pathogens (germs) other than gonorrhea.

Several kinds of pathogens can cause NGU, including:

- *Chlamydia trachomatis*

- *Ureaplasma urealyticum*

- *Trichomonas vaginalis* (rare)

- Herpes simplex virus (rare)

- Adenovirus

- *Haemophilus vaginalis*

- *Mycoplasma genitalium*

NGU is most often caused by chlamydia, a common infection in men and women. The diagnosis of NGU is more commonly made in men than women, primarily due to anatomical differences.

How Is It Transmitted?

Sexual

Most germs that cause NGU can be passed during sex (vaginal, anal, or oral) that involves direct mucous membrane contact with an infected person. These germs can be passed even if the penis or tongue does not go all the way into the vagina, mouth, or rectum, and even if body fluids are not exchanged.

Nonsexual

- Urinary tract infections

- An inflamed prostate gland due to bacteria (bacterial prostatitis)

- A narrowing or closing of the tube in the penis (urethral stricture)

- A tightening of the foreskin so that it cannot be pulled back from the head of the penis (phimosa)

- The result of a process such as inserting a tube into the penis (catheterization)

Perinatal

During birth, infants may be exposed to the germs causing NGU in passage through the birth canal. This may cause the baby to have infections in the:

- eyes (conjunctivitis)

- ears

- lungs (pneumonia)

Symptoms

Men (Urethral Infection)

- Discharge from the penis

- Burning or pain when urinating (peeing)

- Itching, irritation, or tenderness

- Underwear stain

Women (Vaginal/Urethral Infection)

The germs that cause NGU in men might cause other infections in women. These might include vaginitis or mucopurulent cervicitis (MPC). Women may also be asymptomatic (have no symptoms). Symptoms of NGU in women can include:

- Discharge from the vagina

- Burning or pain when urinating (peeing)

- Abdominal pain or abnormal vaginal bleeding may be an indication that the infection has progressed to pelvic inflammatory disease (PID).

Anal or oral infections may result in rectal itching, discharge, or pain on defecation. Most (90 percent) are asymptomatic, but some people might have a sore throat.

Testing/Diagnosis

An NGU diagnosis is made when a man has urethritis (inflammation of the urethra), but gonorrhea is ruled out because he has a negative gonorrhea culture and/or Gram stain. Other tests include: chlamydia culture, urinalysis (sometimes, but rarely). For women: chlamydia culture, gonorrhea culture to rule out gonorrhea.

Treatment

The main treatments for NGU are azithromycin and doxycycline.

Alternatives are erythromycin and ofloxacin.

Recommended treatment for recurrent/persistent urethritis: metronidazole and erythromycin.

A woman who is pregnant, or thinks she might be, should tell her doctor. This will ensure that a medicine will be used that will not harm the baby.

Follow-Up

- Take all medications even if you start to feel better before you finish the bottle.

- Treat all partners.
- Inform all partners.
- Abstain from sex until all partners are treated.
- Return for evaluation by a health care provider if symptoms persist or if symptoms recur after taking all the prescribed medicine.

What Does It Mean For My Health?

Left untreated, the germs that cause NGU, especially chlamydia, can lead to:

Men

- Epididymitis (inflammation of the epididymis, the elongated, cordlike structure along the posterior border of the testes), which can lead to infertility if left, untreated.
- Reiter syndrome (arthritis)
- Conjunctivitis
- Skin lesions
- Discharge

Women

- Pelvic inflammatory disease (PID), which can result in ectopic (tubal) pregnancy.
- Recurrent PID may lead to infertility.
- Chronic pelvic pain
- Urethritis
- Vaginitis
- Mucopurulent cervicitis (MPC)
- Spontaneous abortion (miscarriage)

Men Or Women

- Infections caused by anal sex might lead to severe proctitis (inflamed rectum).

Infants

Exposure to the germs causing NGU during passage through the birth canal may result in infants having:

- Conjunctivitis (If left untreated, this may lead to blindness.)

- Pneumonia

Reduce Your Risk

- Abstinence from sex is the best form of prevention.

- Using latex condoms from start to finish every time you have oral, vaginal, or anal sex.

- Having sex with only one uninfected partner whom only has sex with you (mutual monogamy).

- Water-based spermicides can be used along with latex condoms for additional protection during vaginal intercourse. Use of spermicide is not recommended, nor found to be effective, for oral or anal intercourse.

- Have regular checkups if you are sexually active.

- If you have a sexually transmitted disease (STD), don't have sex (oral, vaginal, anal) until all partners have been treated.

- Prompt, qualified and appropriate medical intervention, treatment, and follow-up are important steps in breaking the disease cycle.

- Know your partner(s). Careful consideration and open communication between partners may protect all partners involved from infection.

Talk To Your Partner

If you have been told that you have NGU, talk to your partner(s), and let them know so they can be tested and treated. The most common cause of NGU is chlamydia, and it is easy to pass from an infected partner to one who is not infected. A man who is diagnosed with NGU should tell his female sex partner and ask her to get tested. He can prevent lasting damage to her body by telling her right away. All sex partners of someone diagnosed with NGU should be treated because:

- They may have an infection and not know it.

- It keeps them from passing the infection back to you or to others.

- It prevents them from suffering possible complications.

☞ Remember!!

Do not have sex until your partner(s) have been tested and treated.

Chapter 69

Pubic Lice

What are pubic lice?

Also called "crabs," pubic lice are parasitic insects found in the genital area of humans. Infection is common and found worldwide.

How did I get pubic lice?

Pubic lice are usually spread through sexual contact. Rarely, infestation can be spread through contact with an infested person's bed linens, towels, or clothes. A common misunderstanding is that infestation can be spread by sitting on a toilet seat. This is not likely, since lice cannot live long away from a warm human body. Also, lice do not have feet designed to walk or hold onto smooth surfaces such as toilet seats.

Where are pubic lice found?

Pubic lice are generally found in the genital area on pubic hair; but may occasionally be found on other coarse body hair, such as hair on the legs, armpits, mustache, beard, eyebrows, or eyelashes. Infestations of young children are usually on the eyebrows or eyelashes. Lice found on the head are not pubic lice; they are head lice.

About This Chapter: Information in this chapter is from "Pubic Lice Infestation," Centers for Disease Control and Prevention, U.S. Department of Health and Human Services, August 2005.

What are the signs and symptoms of pubic lice?

Signs and symptoms of pubic lice include the following:

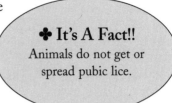

- Itching in the genital area
- Visible nits (lice eggs) or crawling lice

♣ **It's A Fact!!**
Animals do not get or spread pubic lice.

What do pubic lice look like?

There are three stages in the life of a pubic louse: the nit, the nymph, and the adult.

Nit: Nits are pubic lice eggs. They are hard to see and are found firmly attached to the hair shaft. They are oval and usually yellow to white. Nits take about one week to hatch.

Nymph: The nit hatches into a baby louse called a nymph. It looks like an adult pubic louse, but it is smaller. Nymphs mature into adults about seven days after hatching. To live, the nymph must feed on blood.

Adult: The adult pubic louse resembles a miniature crab when viewed through a strong magnifying glass. Pubic lice have six legs, but their two front legs are very large and look like the pincher claws of a crab; this is how they got the nickname "crabs." Pubic lice are tan to grayish-white in color. Females lay nits and are usually larger than males. To live, adult lice must feed on blood. If the louse falls off a person, it dies within one to two days.

How is a pubic lice infestation diagnosed?

A lice infestation is diagnosed by looking closely through pubic hair for nits, nymphs, or adults. It may be difficult to find nymph or adult; there are usually few of them, and they can move quickly away from light. If crawling lice are not seen, finding nits confirms that a person is infested and should be treated. If you are unsure about infestation or if treatment is not successful, see a health care provider for a diagnosis.

How is a pubic lice infestation treated?

A lice-killing shampoo (also called a pediculicide) made of 1% permethrin or pyrethrin is recommended to treat pubic lice. These products are available without a prescription at your local drug store. Medication is generally very effective; apply the medication exactly as directed on the bottle. A prescription medication, called Lindane, is available through your health care provider.

How To Treat Pubic Lice Infestations

The lice medications described in this section should not be used near the eyes.

1. Wash the infested area; towel dry.

2. Thoroughly saturate hair with lice medication. If using permethrin or pyrethrins, leave medication on for ten minutes; if using Lindane, only leave on for four minutes. Thoroughly rinse off medication with water. Dry off with a clean towel.

3. Following treatment, most nits will still be attached to hair shafts. Nits may be removed with fingernails.

4. Put on clean underwear and clothing after treatment.

5. To kill any lice or nits (attached to hairs) that may be left on clothing or bedding, machine wash those washable items that the infested person used during the two to three days before treatment. Use the hot water cycle (130°F). Use the hot dryer cycle for at least 20 minutes.

6. Dry clean clothing that is not washable.

7. Inform any sexual partners that they are at risk for infestation.

8. Do not have sex until treatment is complete.

9. Do not have sex with infected partners until partners have been treated and infestation has been cured.

10. Repeat treatment in seven to ten days if lice are still found.

How To Treat Nits And Lice Found On Eyebrows Or Eyelashes

- If only a few nits are found, it may be possible to remove live lice and nits with your fingernails or a nit comb.

- If additional treatment is needed for pubic lice nits found on the eyelashes, applying an ophthalmic grade petrolatum ointment (only available by prescription) to the eyelids twice a day for ten days is effective. Vaseline is a kind of petrolatum, but it is likely to irritate the eyes if applied.

Chapter 70

Scabies

What is scabies?

Scabies is an infestation of the skin with the microscopic mite *Sarcoptes scabiei*. Infestation is common, found worldwide, and affects people of all races and social classes. Scabies spreads rapidly under crowded conditions where there is frequent skin-to-skin contact between people, such as in hospitals, institutions, childcare facilities, and nursing homes.

What are the signs and symptoms of scabies infestation?

- Pimple-like irritations, burrows or rash of the skin, especially the webbing between the fingers; the skin folds on the wrist, elbow, or knee; the penis, the breast, or shoulder blades

- Intense itching, especially at night and over most of the body

- Sores on the body caused by scratching. These sores can sometimes become infected with bacteria.

How did I get scabies?

People get scabies by direct, prolonged, skin-to-skin contact with a person already infested with scabies. Contact must be prolonged (a quick handshake

About This Chapter: Centers for Disease Control and Prevention, U.S. Department of Health and Human Services, February 2005.

or hug will usually not spread infestation). Infestation may also occur by sharing clothing, towels, and bedding.

Who is at risk for severe infestation?

People with weakened immune systems and the elderly are at risk for a more severe form of scabies, called Norwegian or crusted scabies.

How long will mites live?

Once away from the human body, mites do not survive more than 48–72 hours. When living on a person, an adult female mite can live up to a month.

Did my pet spread scabies to me?

No. Pets become infested with a different kind of scabies mite. If your pet is infested with scabies, (also called mange) and they have close contact with you, the mite can get under your skin and cause itching and skin irritation. However, the mite dies in a couple of days and does not reproduce. The mites may cause you to itch for several days, but you do not need to be treated with special medication to kill the mites. Until your pet is successfully treated, mites can continue to burrow into your skin and cause you to have symptoms.

How soon after infestation will symptoms begin?

For a person who has never been infested with scabies, symptoms may take four to six weeks to begin. For a person who has had scabies, symptoms appear within several days. You do not become immune to an infestation.

How is scabies infestation diagnosed?

Diagnosis is most commonly made by looking at the burrows or rash. A skin scraping may be taken to look for mites, eggs, or mite fecal matter to confirm the diagnosis. If a skin scraping or biopsy is taken and returns negative, it is possible that you may still be infested. Typically, there are fewer than ten mites on the entire body of an infested person; this makes it easy for an infestation to be missed.

Can scabies be treated?

Yes. Several lotions are available to treat scabies. Always follow the directions provided by your physician or the directions on the package insert. Apply lotion to a clean body from the neck down to the toes and left overnight (eight hours). After eight hours, take a bath or shower to wash off the lotion. Put on clean clothes. All clothes, bedding, and towels used by the infested person two days before treatment should be washed in hot water; dry in a hot dryer. A second treatment of the body with the same lotion may be necessary seven to ten days later. Pregnant women and children are often treated with milder scabies medications.

Who should be treated for scabies?

Anyone who is diagnosed with scabies, as well as his or her sexual partners and persons who have close, prolonged contact to the infested person should also be treated. If your health care provider has instructed family members to be treated, everyone should receive treatment at the same time to prevent reinfestation.

How soon after treatment will I feel better?

Itching may continue for two to three weeks and does not mean that you are still infested. Your health care provider may prescribe additional medication to relieve itching if it is severe. No new burrows or rashes should appear 24–48 hours after effective treatment.

Chapter 71

Syphilis

What is syphilis?

Syphilis is a sexually transmitted disease (STD) caused by the bacterium *Treponema pallidum*. It has often been called "the great imitator" because so many of the signs and symptoms are indistinguishable from those of other diseases.

How common is syphilis?

In the United States, health officials reported over 32,000 cases of syphilis in 2002, including 6,862 cases of primary and secondary (P&S) syphilis. The incidence of infectious syphilis was highest in women 20 to 24 years of age and in men 35 to 39 years of age.

Between 2001 and 2002, the number of reported P&S syphilis cases increased 12.4 percent. Rates in women continued to decrease, and overall, the rate in men was 3.5 times that in women. This, in conjunction with reports of syphilis outbreaks in men who have sex with men (MSM), suggests that rates of syphilis in MSM are increasing.

About This Chapter: Centers for Disease Control and Prevention, U.S. Department of Health and Human Services, May 2004.

✤ It's A Fact!!

Syphilis cannot be spread through contact with toilet seats, doorknobs, swimming pools, hot tubs, bathtubs, shared clothing, or eating utensils.

How do people get syphilis?

Syphilis is passed from person to person through direct contact with a syphilis sore. Sores occur mainly on the external genitals, vagina, anus, or in the rectum. Sores also can occur on the lips and in the mouth. Transmission of the organism occurs during vaginal, anal, or oral sex. Pregnant women with the disease can pass it to the babies they are carrying.

What are the signs and symptoms?

Many people infected with syphilis do not have any symptoms for years, yet remain at risk for late complications if they are not treated. Although transmission appears to occur from persons with sores who are in the primary or secondary stage, many of these sores are unrecognized. Thus, most transmission is from persons who are unaware of their infection.

Primary Stage: The primary stage of syphilis is usually marked by the appearance of a single sore (called a chancre), but there may be multiple sores. The time between infection with syphilis and the start of the first symptom can range from 10 to 90 days (average 21 days). The chancre is usually firm, round, small, and painless. It appears at the spot where syphilis entered the body. The chancre lasts three to six weeks, and it heals without treatment. However, if adequate treatment is not administered, the infection progresses to the secondary stage.

Secondary Stage: Skin rash and mucous membrane lesions characterize the secondary stage. This stage typically starts with the development of a rash on one or more areas of the body. The rash usually does not cause itching. Rashes associated with secondary syphilis can appear as the chancre is healing or several weeks after the chancre has healed. The characteristic rash of secondary syphilis may appear as rough, red, or reddish brown spots both on the palms of the hands and the bottoms of the feet. However, rashes with a different appearance may occur on other parts of the body, sometimes resembling rashes caused by other diseases. Sometimes rashes associated with secondary syphilis are so faint that they are not noticed. In addition to rashes, symptoms of secondary syphilis may include fever, swollen lymph glands, sore throat, patchy hair loss, headaches, weight loss, muscle aches, and fatigue. The signs and symptoms of secondary syphilis will resolve with or without treatment; but without treatment, the infection will progress to the latent and late stages of disease.

Late Stage: The latent (hidden) stage of syphilis begins when secondary symptoms disappear. Without treatment, the infected person will continue to have syphilis even though there are no signs or symptoms; infection remains in the body. In the late stages of syphilis, it may subsequently damage the internal organs, including the brain, nerves, eyes, heart, blood vessels, liver, bones, and joints. This internal damage may show up many years later. Signs and symptoms of the late stage of syphilis include difficulty coordinating muscle movements, paralysis, numbness, gradual blindness, and dementia. This damage may be serious enough to cause death.

How is syphilis diagnosed?

Some health care providers can diagnose syphilis by examining material from a chancre (infectious sore) using a special microscope called a darkfield microscope. If syphilis bacteria are present in the sore, they will show up when observed through the microscope.

A blood test is another way to determine whether someone has syphilis. Shortly after infection occurs, the body produces syphilis antibodies that can be detected by an accurate, safe, and inexpensive blood test. A low level of antibodies will stay in the blood for months or years even after the disease has been successfully treated. Because untreated syphilis in a pregnant woman can infect and possibly kill her developing baby, every pregnant woman should have a blood test for syphilis.

What is the link between syphilis and human immunodeficiency virus (HIV)?

Genital sores (chancres) caused by syphilis make it easier to transmit and acquire HIV infection sexually. There is an estimated two- to five-fold increased risk of acquiring HIV infection when syphilis is present.

Ulcerative STDs that cause sores, ulcers, or breaks in the skin or mucous membranes, such as syphilis, disrupt barriers that provide protection against infections. The genital ulcers caused by syphilis can bleed easily, and when they come into contact with oral and rectal mucosa during sex, increase the infectiousness of and susceptibility to HIV. Having other STDs is also an important predictor for becoming HIV infected because STDs are a marker for behaviors associated with HIV transmission.

What is the treatment for syphilis?

Syphilis is easy to cure in its early stages. A single intramuscular injection of penicillin, an antibiotic, will cure a person who has had syphilis for less than a year. Additional doses are needed to treat someone who has had syphilis for longer than a year. For people who are allergic to penicillin, other antibiotics are available to treat syphilis. There are no home remedies or over-the-counter drugs that will cure syphilis. Treatment will kill the syphilis bacterium and prevent further damage, but it will not repair damage already done.

Because effective treatment is available, it is important that persons be screened for syphilis on an on-going basis if their sexual behaviors put them at risk for STDs.

Persons who receive syphilis treatment must abstain from sexual contact with new partners until the syphilis sores are completely healed.

Will syphilis recur?

Having syphilis once does not protect a person from getting it again. Following successful treatment, people can still be susceptible to re-infection. Only laboratory tests

♣ It's A Fact!!
Persons with syphilis must notify their sex partners so that they also can be tested and receive treatment if necessary.

can confirm whether someone has syphilis. Because syphilis sores can be hidden in the vagina, rectum, or mouth, it may not be obvious that a sex partner has syphilis. Talking with a health care provider will help to determine the need to be re-tested for syphilis after treatment has been received.

How can syphilis be prevented?

The surest way to avoid transmission of sexually transmitted diseases, including syphilis, is to abstain from sexual contact or to be in a long-term mutually monogamous relationship with a partner who has been tested and is known to be uninfected.

Genital ulcer diseases, like syphilis, can occur in both male and female genital areas that are covered or protected by a latex condom, as well as in areas that are not covered. Correct and consistent use of latex condoms can reduce the risk of syphilis, as well as genital herpes and chancroid, only when the infected area or site of potential exposure is protected.

Chapter 72

Trichomoniasis

What is trichomoniasis?

Trichomoniasis is a common sexually transmitted disease (STD) that affects both women and men, although symptoms are more common in women.

How common is trichomoniasis?

Trichomoniasis is the most common curable STD in young, sexually active women. An estimated 7.4 million new cases occur each year in women and men.

How do people get trichomoniasis?

Trichomoniasis is caused by the single-celled protozoan parasite, *Trichomonas vaginalis*. The vagina is the most common site of infection in women, and the urethra (urine canal) is the most common site of infection in men. The parasite is sexually transmitted through penis-to-vagina intercourse or vulva-to-vulva (the genital area outside the vagina) contact with an infected partner. Women can acquire the disease from infected men or women, but men usually contract it only from infected women.

About This Chapter: Centers for Disease Control and Prevention, U.S. Department of Health and Human Services, May 2004.

What are the signs and symptoms of trichomoniasis?

Most men with trichomoniasis do not have signs or symptoms; however, some men may temporarily have an irritation inside the penis, mild discharge, or slight burning after urination or ejaculation.

Some women have signs or symptoms of infection, which include a frothy, yellow-green vaginal discharge with a strong odor. The infection also may cause discomfort during intercourse and urination, as well as irritation and itching of the female genital area. In rare cases, lower abdominal pain can occur. Symptoms usually appear in women within 5 to 28 days of exposure.

What are the complications of trichomoniasis?

The genital inflammation caused by trichomoniasis can increase a woman's susceptibility to human immunodeficiency virus (HIV) infection if she is exposed to the virus. Having trichomoniasis may increase the chance that an HIV-infected woman passes HIV to her sex partner(s).

How is trichomoniasis diagnosed?

For both men and women, a health care provider must perform a physical examination and laboratory test to diagnose trichomoniasis. The parasite is harder to detect in men than in women. In women, a pelvic examination can reveal small red ulcerations (sores) on the vaginal wall or cervix.

What is the treatment for trichomoniasis?

Trichomoniasis can usually be cured with the prescription drug, metronidazole, given by mouth in a single dose. The symptoms of trichomoniasis in infected men may disappear within a few weeks without treatment. However, an infected man, even a man who has never had symptoms or whose symptoms have stopped, can continue to infect or re-infect a female partner until he has been treated. Therefore, both partners should be treated at the same

> ♣ **It's A Fact!!**
> Having trichomoniasis once does not protect a person from getting it again. Following successful treatment, people can still be susceptible to re-infection.

time to eliminate the parasite. Persons being treated for trichomoniasis should avoid sex until they and their sex partners complete treatment and have no symptoms.

How can trichomoniasis be prevented?

The surest way to avoid transmission of sexually transmitted diseases is to abstain from sexual contact or to be in a long-term mutually monogamous relationship with a partner who has been tested and is known to be uninfected.

Latex male condoms, when used consistently and correctly, can reduce the risk of transmission of trichomoniasis.

Any genital symptom such as discharge or burning during urination or an unusual sore or rash should be a signal to stop having sex and to consult a health care provider immediately. A person diagnosed with trichomoniasis (or any other STD) should receive treatment and should notify all recent sex partners so that they can see a health care provider and be treated. This reduces the risk that the sex partners will develop complications from trichomoniasis and reduces the risk that the person with trichomoniasis will become re-infected.

Part Seven

If You Need More Information

Chapter 73

Resources For Additional Information About Sexual Development And Sexually Transmitted Diseases

Adolescent AIDS Program

Children's Hospital at Montefiore
Medical Center
111 East 210th Street
Bronx, NY 10467
Phone: 718-882-0232
Fax: 718-882-0432
Website: http://
www.adolescentaids.org
E-mail: info@adolescentaids.org

Advocates For Youth

2000 M Street NW
Suite 750
Washington, DC 20036
Phone: 202-419-3420
Fax: 202-419-1448
Website:
http://www.advocatesforyouth.org

American Academy of Family Physicians

11400 Tomahawk Creek Parkway
Leawood, KS 66211-2672
Toll Free: 800-274-2237
Phone: 913-906-6000
Website:
http://www.aafp.org
E-mail: fp@aafp.org

American Academy of Pediatrics
141 Northwest Point Boulevard
Elk Grove Village, IL 60007-1098
Phone: 847-434-4000
Fax: 847-434-8000
Website: http://www.aap.org

American Board of Obstetrics and Gynecology
2915 Vine Street
Dallas, TX 75204
Phone: 214-871-1619
Fax: 214-871-1943
Website: http://www.abog.org
E-mail: info@abog.org

American College of Obstetricians and Gynecologists (ACOG)
409 12th Street SW
P.O. Box 96920
Washington, DC 20090-6920
Phone: 202-638-5577
Website: http://www.acog.org

American Pregnancy Association
1425 Greenway Drive, Suite 440
Irving, TX 75038
Toll Free: 800-672-2296
Fax: 972-550-0800
Website: http://
www.americanpregnancy.org
E-mail:
Questions@AmericanPregnancy.org

American Psychological Association
750 First Street, NE
Washington, DC 20002-4242
Toll Free: 800-374-2721
Phone: 202-336-5500
TDD/TTY: 202-336-6123
Website: http://www.apa.org

American Social Health Association
P.O. Box 13827
Research Triangle Park, NC 27709
Phone: 919-361-8400
Fax: 919-361-8425
Website: http://www.ashastd.org
Teen-oriented website: http://
www.iwannaknow.org

Association of Reproductive Health Professionals (ARHP)
2401 Pennsylvania Avenue, NW,
Suite 350
Washington, DC 20037-1718
Phone: 202-466-3825
Fax: 202-466-3826
Website: www.arhp.org

Breastcancer.org
111 Forrest Avenue 1R
Narbeth, PA 19072
Website: http://
www.breastcancer.org

Center for Adolescent Health

Johns Hopkins Bloomberg School
of Public Health
615 North Wolfe Street
Room E4612
Baltimore, MD 21205
Phone: 410-614-3953
Fax: 410-614-3956
Website: http://www.jhsph.edu/
adolescenthealth

Center for Young Women's Health

333 Longwood Avenue
5th Floor
Boston, MA 02115
Phone: 617-355-2994
Website: http://
www.youngwomenshealth.org

Centers for Disease Control and Prevention

1600 Clifton Road
Atlanta, GA 30333
Toll Free: 800-311-3435
Website: http://www.cdc.gov

Endometriosis Association

8585 North 76th Place
Milwaukee, WI 53223
Phone: 414-355-2200
Fax: 414-355-6065
Website: http://
www.endometriosisassn.org

Endometriosis Research Center

630 Ibis Drive
Delray Beach, FL 33444
Toll Free: 800-239-7280
Phone: 561-274-7442
Fax: 561-274-0931
Website: http://
www.endocenter.org
E-mail: askerc@aol.com

Focus Adolescent Services

Phone: 410-341-4216
Website: http://www.focusas.com
E-mail: focusashelp.com

Girls and Boys Town

14100 Crawford Street
Boys Town, NE 68010
Toll Free: 800-448-3000
Phone: 402-498-1300
Fax: 402-498-1348
Website: http://
girlsandboystown.org
E-mail:
Hotline@girlsandboystown.org

Alan Guttmacher Institute

125 Maiden Lane, 7th Floor
New York, NY 10038
Toll Free: 800-355-0244
Phone: 212-248-1111
Fax: 212-248-1951
Website: http://
www.guttmacher.org
E-mail: info@guttmacher.org

Hormone Foundation
8401 Connecticut Avenue
Suite 900
Chevy Chase, MD 20815-5817
Toll Free: 800-HORMONE
Fax: 301-941-0259
Website: http://www.hormone.org
E-mail: hormone@endo-society.org

Henry J. Kaiser Family Foundation
2400 Sand Hill Road
Menlo Park, CA 94025
Phone: 650-854-9400
Fax: 650-854-4800
Website: http://www.kff.org

National Campaign to Prevent Teen Pregnancy
1776 Massachusetts Avenue, NW
Suite 200
Washington, DC 20036
Phone: 202-478-8500
Fax: 202-478-8588
Website: http://
www.teenpregnancy.org
E-mail: campaign@thenc.org

National Cancer Institute
NCI Public Inquires Office
6116 Executive Boulevard
Room 3036A
Bethesda, MD 20892-8322
Toll Free: 800-4-CANCER
(800-422-6237)
TTY: 800-332-8615
Website: http://www.cancer.gov

National Cervical Cancer Coalition (NCCC)
7247 Hayvenhurst Avenue
Suite A-7
Van Nuys, CA 91406
Toll Free: 800-685-5531
Phone: 818-909-3849
Fax: 818-780-8199
Website:
http://www.nccc-online.org
E-mail: info@nccc-online.org

National Family Planning and Reproductive Health Association
1627 K Street, NW
12th Floor
Washington, DC 20006
Phone: 202-293-3114
Website: http://www.nfprha.org
E-mail: info@nfprha.org

National Institute of Allergy and Infectious Diseases
NIAID Office of Communications
and Public Liaison
6610 Rockledge Drive
MSC 6612
Bethesda, MD 20892-6612
Phone: 301-496-5717
TDD: 800-877-8339
Fax: 301-402-3573
Website: http://www.niaid.nih.gov

National Institute of Child Health and Human Development (NICHD)

31 Center Drive
Bldg. 31, Room 2A32
MSC 2425
Bethesda, MD 20892-2425
Toll Free: 800-370-2943
Fax: 301-984-1473
TTY: 888-320-6942
Website:
http://www.nichd.nih.gov

National Kidney Foundation

30 East 33rd Street
New York, NY 10016
Toll Free: 800-622-9010
Phone: 212-889-2210
Fax: 212-689-9261
Website: http://www.kidney.org
E-mail: info@kidney.org

National Kidney and Urologic Diseases Information Clearinghouse

3 Information Way
Bethesda, MD 20892-3580
Toll Free: 800-891-5390
Fax: 703-738-4929
Website:
http://kidney.niddk.nih.gov
E-mail:
nkudic@info.niddk.nih.gov

National Prevention Information Network

P.O. Box 6003
Rockville, MD 20849-6003
Toll Free: 800-458-5231
Fax: 888-282-7681
Website: http://cdcnpin.org
E-mail: info@cdcnpin.org

National Women's Health Information Center

U.S. Department of Health and Human Services
8270 Willow Oaks Corporate Drive
Fairfax, VA 22031
Phone: 800-994-9662
TDD: 888-220-5446
Website: http://
www.womenshealth.gov/Pregnancy

Nemours Foundation

Website: http://www.kidshealth.org
E-mail: info@kidshealth.org

Planned Parenthood Federation of America

434 West 33rd Street
New York, NY 10001
Toll-Free: 1-800-230-PLAN
(7526)
Phone: 212-541-7800
Fax: 212-245-1845
Website: http://
www.plannedparenthood.org

STDWeB.com

Wellnet Plaza
5517 State Road
Cleveland, OH 44134
Phone: 888-674-3267
Fax: 440-372-0758
Website: http://www.stdweb.com
E-mail: ask@STDWeB.com

Sexuality Information and Education Council of the United States (SIECUS)

130 West 42nd Street
Suite 350
New York, NY 10036-7802
Phone: 212-819-9770
Fax: 212-819-9776
Website: http://www.siecus.org
E-mail: siecus@siecus.org

Social Health Education

7162 Reading Road
Suite 702
Cincinnati, OH 45237
Phone: 513-924-1444
Fax: 513-924-1434
Website: http://
www.socialhealtheducation.org

tSTD Services Group Inc.

10 South Riverside Plaza
Suite 1800
Chicago, IL 60606
Phone: 888-439-5118
Website: http://www.tstd.org
E-mail: info@tstd.org

U.S. Department of Health and Human Services (HHS)

200 Independence Avenue, SW
Washington, DC 20201
Toll Free: 877-696-6775
Phone: 202-619-0257
Website: http://www.hhs.gov

U.S. Food and Drug Administration (FDA)

5600 Fishers Lane
Rockville, MD 20857
Toll Free: 888-INFO-FDA
(888-463-6332)
Website: http://www.fda.gov

Chapter 74

Additional Reading About Sexuality And Sexual Health

Books

American Medical Association Boy's Guide to Becoming a Teen
Published by Jossey-Bass, May 2006
ISBN: 978-0787983437

American Medical Association Girl's Guide to Becoming a Teen
Published by Jossey-Bass, May 2006
ISBN: 978-0787983444

Date Violence
By Elaine Landau
Published by Franklin Watts, 2004
ISBN: 978-053-1166130

About This Chapter: This chapter includes a compilation of various resources from many sources deemed reliable. It serves as a starting point for further research and is not intended to be comprehensive. Inclusion does not constitute endorsement. Resources in this chapter are categorized by type and, under each type, they are listed alphabetically by title to make topics easier to identify.

Early Puberty in Girls: The Essential Guide to Coping with This Common Problem
By Paul Kaplowitz, M.D., Ph.D.
Published by Ballantine Books, February 2004
ISBN: 978-0345463883

GLBTQ: The Survival Guide for Queer and Questioning Teens
By Kelly Huegel
Published by Free Spirit Publishing, Inc., 2003
ISBN: 978-1575421261

Masturbation as a Means of Achieving Sexual Health
By Walter O. Bockting, Ph.D. and Eli Coleman, Ph.D. (Editors)
Published by The Haworth Press, 2002
ISBN: 978-0789020475

Puberty Survival Guide for Girls
By Dr. Eve Anne Ashby
Published by iUniverse, Inc., February 2005
ISBN: 978-0595342204

The Real Truth About Teens and Sex: From Hooking Up to Friends with Benefits—What Teens Are Thinking, Doing, and Talking About, and How to Help Them Make Smart Choices
By Sabrina Weill
Published by Penguin Group (USA) Inc., September 2006
ISBN: 978-0399532801

S.E.X.: The All-You-Need-To-Know Progressive Sexuality Guide to Get You Through High School and College
By Heather Corinna
Published by Marlow and Company, April 2007
ISBN: 978-1600940101

STDs: What You Don't Know Can Hurt You
By Diane Yancey
Published by Twenty-First Century Books, April 2002
ISBN: 978-0761319573

Safe Sex 101: An Overview for Teens
By Margaret O. Hyde and Elizabeth H. Forsyth, M.D.
Published by Twenty-First Century Books, February 2006
ISBN: 978-0531162125

Sexual Decisions: The Ultimate Teen Guide
By L. Kris Gowen
Published by The Scarecrow Press, May 2007
ISBN: 978-0810858053

Sexually Transmitted Diseases
By Lisa Marr, M.D.
Published by The Johns Hopkins University Press, July 2007
ISBN: 978-0801886591

Sexually Transmitted Infections: The Facts
By David Barlow
Published by Oxford University Press, March 2006
ISBN: 978-0198568674

Teen Rape
By Lynn Slaughter
Published by Lucent Books, March 2004
ISBN: 978-1560065135

The Underground Guide to Teenage Sexuality, 2nd Edition
By Michael J. Basso
Published by Fairview Press, July 2003
ISBN: 978-1577491316

A Woman's Guide to Sexual Health
By Mary Jane Minkin, M.D. and Carol V. Wright, Ph.D.
Published by Yale University Press, 2005
ISBN: 978-0300105940

Articles

"Adolescents' Discussions About Contraception or STDs with Partners Before First Sex," by Suzanne Ryan, Kerry Franzetta, Jennifer Manlove, and Emily Holcombe, *Perspectives on Sexual and Reproductive Health*, September 2007, p. 149(9).

"Advance Provision for Emergency Oral Contraception," by Clarissa Kripke, *American Family Physician*, September 1, 2007, p. 654.

"Banish PMS Forever!" by Melissa Perkins, *Girls' Life*, February-March 2007, p. 50(2).

"Birth Control SOS: The Sex Health Topic You Wonder About Most? Birth Control. So We Rounded Up 10 of Your Most Pressing Contraception Qs—Read On for the Facts," by Marina Khidekel, *CosmoGirl!*, May 2007, p. 86(2).

"Breasts and All the Rest: An Interesting Development," by Ellie Daniels, *New Moon*, November-December 2005, p. 32(2).

"By the Way, Doctor; Is It Safe to Take a Pill That Eliminates Periods?" *Harvard Women's Health Watch*, September 2007, p. NA.

"Conquer Your Gyno-Phobia! Seeing a Gynecologist Sounds Scarier Than It Actually Is—Promise. Here's What Really Goes On Once You Put On That Paper Robe," by Marina Khidekel, *CosmoGirl!*, February 2007, p. 54(2).

"Dear Diary, Yesterday, I Got My Period for the First Time," by Molly Kaye, *New Moon*, July-August 2007, p. 38(2)

"GL Body Q & A," by Kristen Kemp, *Girls' Life*, June-July 2007 v13 i6, p. 30(1).

"Homosexuality and Teens," *Clinical Reference Systems*, May 31, 2007, p. NA.

"Hormone Help: It's Not Just About Birth Control Anymore. New Methods Can Help Manage Heavy Periods, Killer Cramps, PMS, Even Hot Flashes," by Janis Graham, *Good Housekeeping*, June 2007, p. 43(4).

"Know the Facts and Stay Protected: Why You Should Be Practicing Safer Sex," by Shannon Jones, *Ebony*, October 2007, p. 160(2).

"Male Circumcision for Prevention of HIV and Other Sexually Transmitted Diseases," by Patricia Flynn, Peter Havens, Michael Brady, Patricia Emmanuel, Jennifer Read, Laura Hoyt, Lisa Henry-Reid, Russell Van Dyke, and Lynne Mofenson, *Pediatrics*, April 2007, p. 821(2).

"A Mandate in Texas: The Story of a Compulsory Vaccination and What It Means," by Kate O'Beirne, *National Review*, March 5, 2007, p. 18.

"Many Pediatricians Are Reluctant to Vaccinate Young Females Against Human Papillomavirus," by D. Hollander, *Perspectives on Sexual and Reproductive Health*, June 2007, p. 121(2).

"Menstruation in Girls and Adolescents: Using the Menstrual Cycle As a Vital Sign," *Pediatrics*, November 2006, p. 2245(6).

"Myths About Manhood Keep Teen Boys from Sexual Health Care," *Ascribe Higher Education News Service*, April 4, 2007, p. NA.

"New Contraceptives for Women: Dr. Kya Robottom Answers Your Questions About the Latest Advances in Contraceptives," *Ebony*, October 2007, p. 61(1).

"On Guard: Women's Health Activists Are Skeptical About a Federal Plan to Vaccinate Girls as Young as Nine with Gardasil," by Dawn Rae Downton, *Herizons*, Fall 2007, p. 21(4).

"Question Authority: Everything You Wanted to Know but Were Afraid to Ask," by Barbara Homeier, *New Moon*, July-August 2006, p. 38(2).

"Sexual Abstinence," *Clinical Reference Systems*, May 31, 2007, p. NA.

"The Sneaky Threat to Your Fertility: If Caught in Time, Chlamydia Is Harmless. But Left Untreated, This Incredibly Common STD Can Ruin Your Chances of Having Kids One Day. The Worst Part: It's Usually Symptom Free, So You Can't Even Tell You've Been Infected. Cosmo Compiles the Must-Read Facts," by Stacey Colino, *Cosmopolitan*, April 2007, p. 273(4).

"What's Normal Down There? Your Private Parts Are So Mysterious That What Seems Off Can Actually Be Normal. Here's the Good, the Bad, and the Too Embarrassing to Ask," by Marina Khidekel, *CosmoGirl!*, March 2007, p. 95(1).

Index

Index

Page numbers that appear in *Italics* refer to illustrations. Page numbers that have a small 'n' after the page number refer to information shown as Notes at the beginning of each chapter. Page numbers that appear in **Bold** refer to information contained in boxes on that page (except Notes information at the beginning of each chapter).

A

AAFP *see* American Academy of Family Physicians
Abramson, Jon 368
"Abstinence" (American Pregnancy Association) 79n
abstinence (sexual)
  coping strategies **80**
  overview 79–82
abstinence-only education, described **250–54**
acne, puberty 2
ACOG *see* American College of Obstetricians and Gynecologists
acquired immune deficiency syndrome (AIDS)
  circumcision 219
  overview 355–61
ACTH *see* adrenocorticotropin
A.D.A.M., Inc., circumcision publication 217n
Addison disease, described 14
adefovir 352
ADH *see* antidiuretic hormone
Adolescent AIDS Program, contact information 401
adolescent specialists, described **146**

adrenal cortex, described 13–14
adrenal glands, described 13–14
adrenaline *see* epinephrine
adrenal medulla, described 13–14
adrenocorticotropin (ACTH), described 10
advertising, sexuality 101–5
Advocates for Youth
  clinics publication 55n
  contact information 401
age factor
  breast cancer 165
  breast implants **170**
  endometriosis 196
  menstruation **129**
  Pap test 151–53
  pelvic inflammatory disease **190**
  puberty **18**
  testicular cancer **228**
  testicular examination **226**
age of consent, sexual activity 71–72
AIDS *see* acquired immune deficiency syndrome
alcohol use
  breast cancer 166
  date rape 107–8
  sexually transmitted diseases **332–33**

aldosterone, adrenal cortex 13
amenorrhea
    defined **134**
    described 129
    overview 131–32
"Amenorrhea" (NICHD) 127n
American Academy of Family
    Physicians (AAFP), contact
    information 401
American Academy of Pediatrics,
    contact information 402
American Board of Obstetrics and
    Gynecology, contact information
    402
American College of Obstetricians
    and Gynecologists (ACOG),
    contact information 402
American Pregnancy Association
    abstinence publication, 79n
    contact information 402
American Psychological Association,
    contact information 402
American Social Health Association
    (ASHA)
    contact information 402
    nongonococcal urethritis publication
    375n
American Society of Health-System
    Pharmacists (ASHP), vaginal ring
    publication 309n
"Am I ready for sex?" (AVERT) 69n
Anderson, Ralph 368
anorexia nervosa, described 27
"An Overview of Molluscum
    Contagiosum" (CDC) 371n
antidiuretic hormone (ADH),
    described 11
areola 125, 163
ARHP see Association of Reproductive
    Health Professionals
ASHA see American Social Health
    Association
ASHP see American Society of Health-
    System Pharmacists
Association of Reproductive Health
    Professionals (ARHP), contact
    information 402
AVERT, sex readiness publication 69n
azithromycin 377

B

bacterial vaginosis (BV)
    causes **185**
    douching 142
    overview 184–87
"Bacterial Vaginosis" (NWHIC) 181n
"Basics" (VA) 349n
bicuspid aortic valves 203
binge eating, described 27
biopsy
    Pap test 156
    testicular cancer 229–30
birth control
    barrier method 261
    clinics 56
    periodic abstinence 79
    statistics 62–64
    see also pregnancy prevention
birth control pills see oral contraceptives
"Birth Control: Rhythm Method"
    (Nemours Foundation) 257n
bisexuality
    described 91
    HIV infection 95–96
bladder (urinary), defined **178**
blogging, safety considerations 113–15
body changes
    girls 26–27
    puberty 19–23
"Body Hair" (NWHIC) 25n
body odor, puberty 21, 32–33
boner see erections
boys
    enlarged breasts 237–38
    precocious puberty 36–37
    puberty 19–21, 29–34
"Boys and Puberty" (Nemours
    Foundation) 29n
Boys Town see Girls and Boys Town
breast cancer
    combined-hormone contraception **293**
    Depo-Provera injections **300**
    overview 163–67
Breastcancer.org, contact information 402
breast examinations
    cancer screening 157
    described 58
    see also breast self-examination

breast implant surgery, overview 169–71
breasts
    gynecomastia 237–38
    puberty 19, 27–28
    see also mammary glands
breast self-examination (BSE)
    depicted *158–61*
    overview 157–62
    puberty 28
    recommendations **158**
*Breast Self-Examination: Do It
    For Yourself* (State of California) 157n
BSE *see* breast self-examination
bulbourethral glands 215
bulimia nervosa, described 27
butoconazole 183

C

calcium, parathyroid glands 14
cancer
    described 163–64
    HIV infection 361
Candida 181
CDC *see* Centers for Disease
    Control and Prevention
cells of Leydig 211
Center for Adolescent Health, contact
    information 403
Center for Young Women's Health,
    contact information 403
Centers for Disease Control and
    Prevention (CDC)
    contact information 403
    publications
        chlamydia 335n
        molluscum contagiosum 371n
        pelvic inflammatory disease 189n
        pubic lice 381n
central precocious puberty 35–36
cervical cancer
    human papillomavirus 364
    Pap test 153
    risk factors **365**
"Cervical Cancer Vaccine
    Continues to Spark Debate"
    (NWHIC) 363n
cervical caps, described 271–79
cervical shields, described 271–79

cervix
    depicted *120*
    Pap test 151
"Changes to Your Breast" (NWHIC) 25n
"Changes to Your Mind" (NWHIC) 25n
"Changes to Your Shape" (NWHIC) 25n
chat rooms
    permission **112**
    safety considerations 112–13
chemotherapy, testicular cancer 231–32
chlamydia, overview 335–38
"Chlamydia - CDC Fact Sheet" (CDC)
    335n
Chlamydia trachomatis 335, 375
chromosomes
    defined **126**
    delayed puberty 41–42
    Klinefelter syndrome **41**, 239
    oogenesis 120–21
    spermatogenesis 211
    Turner syndrome **41**
Cincinnati Children's Hospital Medical
    Center, precocious puberty publication 35n
circumcision
    overview 217–20
    parental decisions **219**
"Circumcision" (A.D.A.M., Inc.) 217n
clindamycin 186
"Clinical Features of Turner
    Syndrome" (NICHD) 201n
clinics, overview 55–59
clitoris
    depicted *120*, *124*
    described 124
clotrimazole 183
coarctation of aorta 203
colposcopy, described 155–56
coming out, described 94–95
communication
    sex discussions 65–67
    sexual health 52
condoms
    benefits **264**
    chlamydia 338
    gonorrhea 348
    oral sex 88
    overview 261–66
    proper usage **262–63**
    trichomoniasis 397

contraceptives, continuous use drug 286–87
contraceptive sponges
  described 282
  overview 281–82
conversion therapies, homosexuality 92–93
Cooper's ligaments 126
corona radiata 122
corpora cavernosa 216
corpus albicans 122
corpus luteum 122, 125
corpus spongiosum 216
cortex 120
cortisol
  adrenal cortex 13, 14
  described 10
counseling
  homosexuality 92–93
  pregnancy tests 56–57
  transgendered persons 99
Cowper glands
  depicted 210
  described 215
crabs see pubic lice
cremaster muscle 210
Cushing syndrome, described 14
cystoscope 178

D

dartos muscle 210
date rape, overview 107–9
date rape drugs, described 107–8
"Delayed Puberty" (Nemours
  Foundation) 39n
delayed puberty, overview 39–43
Department of Health and Human
  Services see US Department of Health
  and Human Services
Depo-Provera, overview 299–301
"Depo-Provera Injections" (Women's
  College Hospital) 299n
DHHS see US Department of
  Health and Human Services
diabetes mellitus
  insulin 15
  Turner syndrome 204
diaphragms
  described 271–79
  toxic shock syndrome 276

"Diaphragms, Caps, and Shields" (PPFA)
  271n
diet and nutrition, puberty 30
"Do I Need to See a Gynecologist?"
  (NWHIC) 145n
douching
  bacterial vaginosis 185, 187
  overview 141–44
  pelvic inflammatory disease 190
  recommendations 143
Down syndrome, Turner syndrome 204
doxycycline 377
DUB see dysfunctional uterine bleeding
ductus deferens see vas deferens
dysfunctional uterine bleeding
  (DUB) 130
dysmenorrhea
  defined 134
  described 129
  overview 133–35
"Dysmenorrhea (Painful Periods)"
  (Washington State University) 127n

E

early puberty see precocious puberty
eating disorders
  delayed puberty 40–41
  puberty 27
ECP see emergency contraceptive pills
ejaculation, described 21, 34, 216
ejaculatory duct, described 213–14
embarrassment, sex discussions 23
emergency contraception, overview
  323–27
emergency contraceptive pills
  (ECP) 324–27
Emory University, tubal ligation
  publication 317n
emotional concerns
  precocious puberty 38
  premenstrual syndrome 137–38
  puberty 21–23, 28, 45–47
  sexual activity 69–71
"Endo 101: The Endocrine System"
  (Hormone Foundation) 7n
endocervical curettage, described 156
"Endocrine Glands" (Hormone
  Foundation) 7n

endocrine glands, described 9, 10–15
endocrine system
    depicted *8*
    described 7–9
endocrinologists
    defined **41**
    delayed puberty 42–43
    described **9**
endometriosis, overview 195–200
Endometriosis Association, contact
    information 403
Endometriosis Research Center,
    contact information 403
endometrium, described 123, 195
enfuvirtide 360–61
entecavir 352
epididymis
    depicted *210*
    described 213
epididymitis, gonorrhea 347
epinephrine (adrenaline), adrenal
    medulla 14
erections
    frequency **34**
    puberty 21, 33–34
    see also penis
erythromycin 377
estrogen
    defined **22, 126**
    described 12
    menstrual cycle 128
    oral contraceptives 283
    Ortho Evra 293
    puberty 126
ethnic factors, hepatitis B vaccine **352**
"Etonogestrel and Ethinyl Estradiol
    Vaginal Ring" (ASHP) 309n
etonogestrel and ethinyl estradiol vaginal
    ring, overview 309–16
eukaryotic organisms, described **126**
"Everything You Wanted to Know About
    Puberty" (Nemours Foundation) 17n
"Examining Oral Sex" (PPFA) 87n
external genitalia, female 124

F

"Facts About Vasectomy Safety" (NICHD)
    317n

"Facts on American Teens' Sexual and
    Reproductive Health" (Guttmacher
    Institute) 61n
fallopian tubes
    described 123
    endometriosis 197, 198
    pelvic inflammatory disease 191
Family Planning Association of
    Western Australia, intrauterine
    devices publication 303n
family practitioners, described **146**
FDA *see* US Food and Drug
    Administration
female condoms, overview 267–69
    see also condoms
female reproductive system
    depicted *120*
    overview 119–26
female sexual response, hormones
    124–25
FemCap *see* cervical caps
fertilization, described 122
fetus, defined **126**
fever blisters, genital herpes 340
fimbriae 123
financial considerations
    birth control **296**
    cervical cancer vaccine 367, 369
    clinics 55–56
    condoms 263
    diaphragms 279
    spermicides 279
fluconazole 183
fluoxetine 140
Focus Adolescent Services,
    contact information 403
follicle stimulating hormone (FSH)
    defined **22**
    described 10, 124–25, 216
    menstruation 128
    puberty 18, 121–22
Food and Drug Administration
    see US Food and Drug
    Administration
foreskin 216, 217
Frenck, Robert 367
FSH *see* follicle stimulating hormone
fusion inhibitors 360–61
Fuzeon 360–61

G

gamma-hydroxybutyrate (GHB) 108
Gardasil 64, 366
gay, described 91
Gelperin, Nora 88–89
gender identity, transgendered
  persons 97–99
general practitioners, described **146**
genes
  personal looks 3–4
  SHOX 201–2
  see also heredity
genital herpes
  overview 339–43
  sexual activity **341**
genitalia
  female *124*
  male *210*
genital warts, human papillomavirus 364
germinal epithelium 120
GH *see* growth hormone
GHB *see* gamma-hydroxybutyrate
girls
  precocious puberty 36
  puberty 19–21, 25–28
  reproductive system overview 119–26
Girls and Boys Town, contact
  information 109, 403
glands, described **10**
glans penis 216
glucagon, pancreas 14
glucocorticoids, adrenal cortex 13
GnRH *see* gonadotropin releasing
  hormone
goiter, described 13
gonadotropin, described 12
gonadotropin dependent
  precocious puberty 35–36
gonadotropin independent
  precocious puberty 36
gonadotropin releasing hormone
  (GnRH)
  defined **22**
  described 17–18
gonads *see* ovaries; testicles
gonorrhea
  overview 345–48
  sexual activity **346**

graafian follicle 122
Greer, Jim 45–46
group A *Streptococcus* 173
growth hormone (GH)
  described 10
  Turner syndrome 202
growth spurt
  girls 26
  overview 3–5
  puberty 18–19
Alan Guttmacher Institute
  contact information 403
  statistics publication 61n
gynecologists
  described **146, 148**
  overview 145–49
gynecomastia
  Klinefelter syndrome **41**
  overview 237–38

H

hair growth
  boys 32
  girls 26
  puberty 20
hardon *see* erections
hate crimes, homosexuality 95
health care
  clinics 55–59
  gynecologists 145–49
  menstruation 130
  pelvic inflammatory disease 192–93
  see also clinics
hepatitis B
  overview 349–53
  prevention **350**
  vaccine **352**
heredity
  body height 30
  breast cancer 165
  delayed puberty 40
  endometriosis **199**
  personal looks 3–4
  precocious puberty 35
  testicular cancer 228
  see also genes
hermaphrodites, described 98
herpes simplex virus (HSV) 339

HHS *see* US Department of Health
  and Human Services
HI *see* hyperinsulinism
HIV infection
  casual contact **357**
  gonorrhea 347
  homosexuality 95–96
  molluscum contagiosum 373
  overview 355–61
  Pap test 152
  prevention **361**
  sexually transmitted diseases 333
  statistics 64
  syphilis 392
"HIV Infection and AIDS:
  An Overview" (NIAID) 355n
homosexuality, overview 91–96
Hormone Foundation, contact
  information 404
hormones
  delayed puberty **42**
  female sexual response 124–25
  gynecomastia 237–38
  menstrual cycle 128
  Ortho Evra 292–93
  overview 7–15
  pituitary gland **22**
  premenstrual syndrome 137
  puberty 17–18
  Turner syndrome 202
hormone therapy, endometriosis 199
HPV *see* human papillomavirus
"HPV (human papillomavirus)"
  (DHHS) 363n
HSV *see* herpes simplex virus
human immunodeficiency virus
  see HIV infection
human papillomavirus (HPV)
  overview 363–69
  Pap test 153–54
  statistics 63–64
humoral factors, described 11
hyperinsulinism (HI), described 15
hyperthyroidism, described 13
hypoglycemia (low blood sugar),
  described 15
hypothalamus
  described 11
  hormones **22**

hypothyroidism
  described 13
  Turner syndrome 204
hysterectomy
  endometriosis 200
  Pap test 153

I

IM *see* instant message
"I'm a Guy... so How Come I'm
  Developing Breasts?" (Nemours
  Foundation) 237n
"I'm Growing Up - But Am I Normal?"
  (Nemours Foundation) 3n
"The Importance of Talking to Your Parents
  About Sex and Sexuality" (Planned
  Parenthood of New York City) 65n
infants
  hypoglycemia 15
  hypothyroidism 13
infundibulum 123
inhibin, described 12
instant message (IM), safety
  considerations 112
insulin, pancreas 14–15
insulinoma, described 15
intercourse *see* sexual activity
interferon 352
internet safety, personal information **114**
internet sexual predators, protection 111–15
intersexed persons, described 98
intrauterine devices (IUD)
  emergency contraception 324–25
  overview 303–8
  pelvic inflammatory disease 190
"Intrauterine Devices and Systems"
  (Family Planning Association of
  Western Australia) 303n
intrauterine systems (IUS) 303–8
IUD *see* intrauterine devices
IUS *see* intrauterine systems

K

Kaiser Family Foundation, virginity
  publication 69n
Henry J. Kaiser Family Foundation,
  contact information 404

Kaposi sarcoma 361
kidney disorders,
    Turner syndrome 203
kidneys, defined **178**
Klinefelter, Henry 239
Klinefelter syndrome
    defined **41**
    described 42
    overview 239–41

L

labia majora *120, 124*
labia minora *120, 124*
lactiferous ducts 126
lamivudine 352
late puberty *see* delayed puberty
latex condoms *see* condoms
lesbians, described 91
lesions, genital herpes 340
LH *see* luteinizing hormone
LHRH *see* luteinizing releasing
    hormone
"Life After Puberty: Masturbation"
    (SOGC) 83n
lobes
    described 163
    mammary glands 126
low blood sugar *see* hypoglycemia
LUMA Cervical Imaging System 156
lumen 211
luteinizing hormone (LH)
    defined **22**
    described 10, 124–25, 216
    menstruation 128
    puberty 18
luteinizing releasing hormone
    (LHRH), precocious puberty **38**
Lybrel, described **286–87**
lymph nodes
    cancer 164
    described 163

M

magnetic resonance imaging (MRI)
    endometriosis 198
    precocious puberty 37
male condoms *see* condoms

male reproductive system
    depicted *210*
    overview 209–16
male sexual response, described 216
mammary glands, described 125–26
    see also breasts
mammograms, cancer screening 157
mass media
    sexuality 101–5
    sexual messages **104**
master gland *see* pituitary gland
masturbation
    described **84**
    overview 83–85
    sexual health 52
Medical Institute for Sexual Health,
    nonmarital pregnancy publication 245n
medications
    bacterial vaginosis 186
    chlamydia 337
    dysmenorrhea 135
    endometriosis 199
    gonorrhea 347–48
    hepatitis B 352
    HIV infection 360–61
    nongonococcal urethritis 377
    premenstrual dysphoric disorder 140
    premenstrual syndrome 139
    pubic lice 382–83
    scabies 387
    syphilis 392
    trichomoniasis 396
    urinary tract infections 178–79
    vaginal yeast infections 183
medulla 120
meiotic division 121, 211–12
melatonin, described 12
menarche, described **129**
menopause, described 12, 125
menorrhagia 130
menses *see* menstruation
menstrual cycle
    described 127–28
    oral contraceptives 284–85
    see also premenstrual syndrome
menstruation
    defined **134**
    endometrium 123
    ovaries 12–13

menstruation, continued
  overview 127–35
  puberty 19–20
  uterine cycle 125
"Menstruation and the Menstrual
  Cycle" (NWHIC) 127n
mental health
  homosexuality 93
  sexual health 53
metastasize, described 164
metronidazole 186, 377, 396
miconazole 183
milk ducts, mammary glands 126
mineralocorticoids,
  adrenal cortex 13
Mirena 303
mitosis 211–12
molluscum contagiosum,
  overview 371–73
mons pubis *120, 124*
mood changes
  premenstrual syndrome 138
  puberty **46**
morning after pill 325
muscles, puberty 30–31

N

National Campaign to Prevent
  Teen Pregnancy, contact
  information 404
National Cancer Institute (NCI)
  contact information 404
  publications
    breast cancer 163n
    female reproductive system 119n
    male reproductive system 209n
    testicular cancer 227n
National Cervical Cancer Coalition
  (NCCC), contact information 404
National Domestic Violence Hotline,
  contact information 109
National Family Planning and
  Reproductive Health Association,
  contact information 404
National Institute of Allergy and
  Infectious Diseases (NIAID)
  contact information 404
  HIV infection publication 355n

National Institute of Child Health and
  Human Development (NICHD)
  contact information 405
  publications
    amenorrhea 127n
    Turner syndrome 201n
    vasectomy 317n
National Institute of Diabetes and
  Digestive and Kidney Diseases
  (NIDDK)
  contact information 405
  urinary tract infections publication 177n
National Kidney Foundation, contact
  information 405
National Prevention Information
  Network, contact information 405
National Sexual Assault Hotline, contact
  information 108, 109
National Women's Health Information
  Center (NWHIC)
  contact information 405
  publications
    bacterial vaginosis 181n
    cervical cancer vaccine 363n
    date rape 107n
    gynecologists 145n
    menstruation 127n
    online sexual predators 111n
    puberty, girls 25n
    sexually transmitted diseases 331n
    vaginal yeast infections 181n
NCCC *see* National Cervical Cancer
  Coalition
NCI *see* National Cancer Institute
Neisseria gonorrhoeae 345
Nemours Foundation
  contact information 405
  publications
    delayed puberty 39n
    growing up 3n
    gynecomastia 237n
    puberty 17n
    puberty, boys 29n
    rhythm method 257n
NGU *see* nongonococcal urethritis
"NGU (Nongonococcal Urethritis):
  Questions and Answers" (ASHA) 375n
NIAID *see* National Institute of Allergy
  and Infectious Diseases

NICHD *see* National Institute of Child Health and Human Development
NIDDK *see* National Institute of Diabetes and Digestive and Kidney Diseases
nipples
    described 163
    mammary glands 125–26
nocturnal emissions
    overview 223–24
    puberty 21, 34
nongonococcal urethritis (NGU), overview 375–80
"Nonmarital Pregnancy" (Medical Institute for Sexual Health) 245n
non-nucleoside reverse transcriptase inhibitors 360
nonoxynol-9
    contraceptive sponges **282**
    sexually transmitted diseases 275
nonseminomas, described 227, 230
norepinephrine, adrenal medulla 14
nurse practitioners, described **146**
NWHIC *see* National Women's Health Information Center
nystatin 183

O

obstetricians, described **148**
ofloxacin 377
online profiles, safety considerations 113–15
online sexual predators, protection 111–15
oocytes 120
oogenesis, described 120–21
opportunistic infections
    described 355
    medications 361
oral contraceptives
    described **284**
    overview 283–88
oral sex
    overview 87–89
    virginity 74
orgasm
    described 83, 216
    fertilization 124
Ortho Evra (the patch),
    overview 289–98

osteoporosis
    Depo-Provera injections **300**
    Turner syndrome 203–4
ovarian follicle development, described 121–22
ovarian fossae 119
ovaries
    depicted *120*
    described 12–13, 19–20, 119–22
    puberty 18
    reproductive system **119, 120**
oviducts 123
ovulation, described 122, 125, 128
ovulation test kits 257, 259
oxytocin
    described 11
    puberty 126

P

pancreas, described 14–15
Pap test
    cervical cancer **152**
    gynecologists 149
    human papillomavirus 366
    overview 151–56
    recommendations **154**
parathyroid glands, described 14
parents
    homosexuality 94
    sex discussions 65–67
paroxetine 140
passwords, safety considerations 112, 115
"The Patch" (PPFA) 289n
the patch *see* Ortho Evra
Paxil (paroxetine) 140
PCOS *see* polycystic ovary syndrome
pediatricians, described **146**
pegylated interferon 352
pelvic examinations
    described 57–58
    gynecologists 148
pelvic inflammatory disease (PID)
    bacterial vaginosis 186
    chlamydia 337
    douching 142
    gonorrhea 347
    overview 189–93

"Pelvic Inflammatory Disease
   - CDC Fact Sheet" (CDC) 189n
penile cancer 218–19
penis
   depicted *210*
   described 216
   overview 221–22
   see also erections
period *see* menstruation
permethrin 382–83
phimosis 218–19
PID *see* pelvic inflammatory disease
the pill *see* oral contraceptives
pimples *see* acne
pineal gland, described 12
pituitary gland
   defined **22**
   delayed puberty 41
   described 10–11
   puberty 17–18
pituitary hormones
   described 11
   underproduction **11**
Plan-B 324–25
Planned Parenthood Federation
   of America (PPFA)
   contact information 405
   publications
      diaphragms 271n
      nocturnal emissions 223n
      oral sex 87n
      patch 289n
      puberty side effects 45n
      sexual health 51n
Planned Parenthood of New York
   City, parental unit discussions
   publication 65n
"Pleasant Dreams! A Guide to
   Nocturnal Emissions" (PPFA) 223n
PMDD *see* premenstrual dysphoric
   disorder
PMS *see* premenstrual syndrome
polycystic ovary syndrome (PCOS),
   described 13
PPFA *see* Planned Parenthood
   Federation of America
precocious puberty
   overview 35–38
   synthetic hormones **38**

"Precocious Puberty (Early Puberty)"
   (Cincinnati Children's Hospital
   Medical Center) 35n
pregnancy
   bacterial vaginosis 186
   douching 144
   overview 245–48
   statistics 64
pregnancy prevention
   abstinence programs 249–56
   cervical shields 271–79
   contraceptive sponges 281–82
   Depo-Provera 299–301
   diaphragms 271–79
   intrauterine devices 303–8
   oral contraceptives 283–88
   Ortho Evra (the patch) 289–98
   rhythm method 257–59
   sterilization 317–22
   vaginal rings 309–16
   see also birth control
pregnancy tests, clinics 56–57
prejudice, homosexuality 95
premenstrual dysphoric disorder
   (PMDD), described 139–40
premenstrual syndrome (PMS)
   overview 137–40
   symptoms **138**
prepuce *124*, 216
primary amenorrhea, described 131, 132
PRL *see* prolactin
progesterone
   described 12
   menstrual cycle 128
   puberty 126
progestin
   Depo-Provera 299–301
   emergency contraception 324–25
   oral contraceptives 283
prokaryotic organisms, described **126**
prolactin (PRL)
   described 10
   puberty 126
prostaglandins, dysmenorrhea 129,
   133–34
prostate gland
   depicted *210*
   described 215
protease inhibitors 360

Province of British Columbia, toxic
  shock syndrome publication 173n
pseudogynecomastia 238
puberty
  age factor **18**
  described 25–26
  growth spurt 4, **5**
  mood changes 45–47
  oocytes 121
  overview 17–23
  sperm production **212**
  temporary breast tissue growth **238**
  Turner syndrome **202**
  see also delayed puberty; precocious
    puberty
"Puberty" (NWHIC) 25n
pubic lice, overview 381–84
"Pubic Lice Infestation" (CDC) 381n
pudendum 124
pyrethrin 382–83

R

radiation therapy, testicular cancer 231
radical inguinal orchiectomy 229, 230–31
rape, overview 107–9
recurrent vulvovaginal candidiasis
  (RVVC) 184
reproductive system
  female 119–26, *120*
  male 209–16, *210*
"Reproductive System" (NCI-SEER)
  119n, 209n
rete testis 211
reverse transcriptase inhibitors 360
rhythm method, described 257–59
risk factors
  breast cancer 165–67
  cervical cancer **365**
  endometriosis 196–97
  hepatitis B 349–50
  testicular cancer 228
RVVC *see* recurrent vulvovaginal
  candidiasis

S

"Safe Blogging" (NWHIC) 111n
"Safe Chatting" (NWHIC) 111n

safer sex, hepatitis B **350**
safe sex
  information 73
  intrauterine devices **305**
safety considerations, online sexual
  predators 111–15
"Safety on the Internet" (NWHIC) 111n
Sager, Jennifer 97n
sanitary pads, menstrual cycle 129, 130–31
  see also tampons
Sarafem (fluoxetine) 140
Sarcoptes scabiei 385
scabies, overview 385–87
"Scientific Evaluations of Approaches
  to Prevent Teen Pregnancy"
  (Solomon-Fears) 249n
scrotum
  depicted *210*
  described 209–10, 227
secondary amenorrhea, described 131,
  132
semen (seminal fluid)
  described 21, 215
  nocturnal emissions 34
seminal vesicles
  depicted *210*
  described 214
seminiferous tubules
  depicted *210*
  described 211
seminomas, described 227, 230
serotonin reuptake inhibitors (SSRI),
  premenstrual dysphoric disorder 140
sertraline 140
"Seven Steps to Sexual Health"
  (PPFA) 51n
sex education, described **252–54**
sex hormones, adrenal cortex 14
"SexSmarts Survey - Virginity and
  The First Time" (Kaiser Family
  Foundation) 69n
sexual abuse, described 53
sexual activity
  delay **76, 78**
  overview 69–78
  statistics 61–62
sexual health
  described **52**
  overview 51–53

Sexuality Information and Education
    Council of the United States (SIECUS)
    contact information 406
"Sexuality in the Mass Media: How to
    View the Media Critically" (University
    of California) 101n
sexually transmitted diseases (STD)
    abstinence 80
    bacterial vaginosis 186
    circumcision 218
    clinics 57
    condoms 265
    contraceptive sponges 282
    douching 142, 144
    female condoms 268–69
    gynecologists 149
    intrauterine devices 305
    oral sex 88, 88
    overview 331–34
    pelvic inflammatory disease 189–90,
        193, 193
    prevention 334
    statistics 63–64
    vaginal ring 310
    vasectomy 321
"Sexually Transmitted Diseases:
    Overview" (NWHIC) 331n
sexual orientation
    described 98
    overview 91–96
sexual predators, protection 111–15
shield see cervical shields
the shot see Depo-Provera
SIECUS see Sexuality Information and
    Education Council of the United States
Social Health Education, contact
    information 406
social networking, safety considerations
    113–15
Society of Obstetricians and
    Gynaecologists of Canada (SOGC),
    masturbation publication 83n
SOGC see Society of Obstetricians
    and Gynaecologists of Canada
Solomon-Fears, Carmen 249n
speculum 148
sperm
    body temperature 209
    fertilization 215

sperm, continued
    formation 211–12
    puberty 34, 212
spermatogenesis, described 211–12
spermicides
    contraceptive sponges 282
    described 262
    sexually transmitted diseases 275
sports, testicular injury 233–36
sports bra 28
spurt, defined 18–19
SSRI see serotonin reuptake
    inhibitors
Staphylococcus aureus 173
State of California, breast self-
    examinations publication 157n
statistics
    AIDS 356
    birth control access 63–64
    breast cancer 167
    breast implant surgery 169
    chlamydia 335
    condom breakage 261
    contraceptive use 62–63
    endometriosis 196
    genital herpes 339
    gonorrhea 345
    HIV infection 356
    Klinefelter syndrome 240
    pelvic inflammatory disease 189
    pregnancy 64
    premenstrual syndrome 138
    sexual activity 61–62, 75, 77–78
    sexually transmitted diseases 331
    syphilis 389
    teen pregnancy 245–48
    television sexual content 102–3
    television watching 101
    testicular cancer 227–28
    trichomoniasis 395
    Turner syndrome 201
    vaginal yeast infections 183
STDWeB.com, contact information
    406
sterilization, overview 317–22
stratum basale 123
stratum functionale 123
stress management, puberty 47
substance abuse, sexual health 53

surgical procedures
  breast implants 169–71
  endometriosis 199–200
  radical inguinal orchiectomy 229,
    230–31
  tubal ligation 317–19
  vasectomy 319–22
"Surviving Puberty: Moods and
  Emotions" (PPFA) 45n
suspensory ligaments 126
symphysis pubis *120*
synthetic hormones, precocious
  puberty **38**
syphilis
  casual contact **390**
  overview 389–93

T

T3 *see* triiodothyronine
T4 *see* thyroxine
T-20 360
tampons
  described 130–31
  quick tips **130**
  toxic shock syndrome **174**, 174–75
  see also sanitary pads
technical virginity, oral sex 74, 87–88
terconazole 183
testes *see* testicles
testicles (testes)
  depicted *210*
  described 12, 209–11, 227
  puberty 18
testicular cancer
  described 12
  early detection **230**
  overview 227–32
"Testicular Cancer: Questions
  and Answers" (NCI) 227n
testicular injury
  overview 233–36
  prevention **236**
testicular rupture 235
"Testicular Self-Exam" (University
  of Ottawa) 225n
testicular self-examination,
  overview 225–26
testicular torsion 234

testosterone
  defined **22**
  described 12
  Klinefelter syndrome **41**, 240–41
  puberty 18
tests
  bacterial vaginosis 185
  chlamydia 337
  delayed puberty 42
  endometriosis 198
  genital herpes 341–42
  gonorrhea 347
  hepatitis B 351
  human papillomavirus 364
  nongonococcal urethritis 377
  precocious puberty 37
  sexually transmitted diseases 332
  syphilis 391
  testicular cancer 229–30
  trichomoniasis 396
  vaginal ring **316**
  see also Pap test
thymus, described 11
thyroid gland
  delayed puberty 41
  described 13
thyroid stimulating hormone (TSH),
  described 10
thyroxine (T4), described 13
tioconazole 183
tobacco use, vaginal ring **313**
"Toxic Shock Syndrome" (Province
  of British Columbia) 173n
toxic shock syndrome (TSS)
  described 131
  diaphragms **276**
  overview 173–75
transgendered persons, overview 97–99
transsexuals, described 97
transvestites, described 98
Treponema pallidum 389
Trichomonas vaginalis 395
trichomoniasis
  infection 331
  overview 395–97
  reinfection **396**
triiodothyronine (T3), described 13
TSH *see* thyroid stimulating hormone
TSS *see* toxic shock syndrome

tSTD Services Group Inc., contact
   information 406
tubal ligation
   defined 322
   overview 317–19
"Tubal Ligation" (Emory University) 317n
tumor markers, testicular cancer 229
tumors, described 164
tunica albuginea 120, 211
Turner syndrome
   defined 41
   described 41–42
   overview 201–5
   puberty 202
two spirited, described 98

U

ultrasound
   endometriosis 198
   precocious puberty 37
   testicular cancer 229
"Understanding Transgender" (Sager) 97n
University of California, mass media,
   sexuality publication 101n
University of Ottawa, testicular self-
   examination publication 225n
ureter, defined 178
urethra
   defined 178
   described 34, 214
   female 120
   male 214
urinary tract infections (UTI), overview
   177–80
US Department of Health and Human
   Services (DHHS; HSS)
   contact information 406
   human papillomavirus publication 363n
US Department of Veterans Affairs (VA),
   hepatitis B publication 349n
US Food and Drug Administration (FDA),
   contact information 406
uterine bleeding, described 130
uterine cycle, described 125
uterus
   depicted 120, 123
   described 123
UTI see urinary tract infections

V

VA see US Department
   of Veterans Affairs
vaccines
   cervical cancer 367–69
   hepatitis B 350, 352–53
   human papillomavirus 366–67
vagina
   depicted 120, 124
   described 123–24, 125
   douching 141–43
vaginal rings, overview 309–16
"Vaginal Yeast Infections"
   (NWHIC) 181n
vaginal yeast infections,
   overview 181–84
valacyclovir 342
Valtrex (valacyclovir) 342
vas deferens
   depicted 210
   described 213
vasectomy
   defined 322
   overview 319–22
vesicular follicle 122
vestibule 124
viral hepatitis, described 349
virginity
   described 74
   first sexual encounter 74–77
   oral sex 74, 87–88
voice changes, puberty 19, 21
vulva 124

W

Washington State University,
   dysmenorrhea publication 127n
weight gain, puberty 19
weight lifting, recommendations
   30–31
wet dreams
   overview 223–24
   puberty 21, 34
   stress 224
"What I Need to Know about
   Urinary Tract Infections"
   (NIDDK) 177n

"What is rape and date rape?" (NWHIC) 107n

"What You Need To Know About Breast Cancer" (NCI) 163n

Women's College Hospital, Depo-Provera injections publication 299n

Wright, Wendy 369

X

XXY males 239–41
  see also Klinefelter syndrome

Y

yeast infections, overview 181–84

"Your Growth Spurt" (NWHIC) 25n

"Your Guide to the Clinic" (Advocates for Youth) 55n

Z

zits *see* acne

Zoloft (sertraline) 140

zona pellucida 122